4.95

Anthony J. Gammell

Swatcol
at 'EBBA's'
Byam
Surrey

HANDBOOK
OF
INVESTIGATIONS

HANDBOOK OF INVESTIGATIONS

Edited by

Jennifer A Booth, SRN, SCM, RNT, Dip.Ed

formerly Senior Tutor to the SRN/DN Course
now Senior Tutor (Postbasic Education)
Macdonald Buchanan School of Nursing
The Middlesex Hospital
London

Harper & Row, Publishers
London

Cambridge
Hagerstown
Philadelphia
New York

San Francisco
Mexico City
Sao Paulo
Sydney

Copyright © 1983 JA Booth
All rights reserved
First published 1983. Reprinted 1983, 1986
Harper & Row Ltd
28 Tavistock Street
London WC2E 7PN

British Library cataloguing in Publication Data

Nurses handbook of investigations.
   1. Physical diagnosis   2. Nursing
   I. Booth, Jenny
   616.07′54′024613   RC76

   ISBN 0-06-318235-1

Typeset by *Sunrise Setting*, Torquay, Devon
Printed and bound by The Bath Press, Avon

CONTRIBUTORS

Gillian Auger
Christine Barker
Ann Benson
Gillian Branch
Shona Davison
Christine Dewey
Annette Hitchings
Janet Holden
Karen Howard-Luck
Rachel Butterfield
Penny White

Third year students undertaking a 199-week course leading to State Registration and the Diploma in Nursing (London University).

CONTENTS

ACKNOWLEDGMENTS

We would like to thank all the ward, medical and departmental staff at the Middlesex Hospital who made the initial project and this book possible. Without their encouragement and enthusiasm this text would not have been produced.

Thanks must also go to the patients who made us aware of the need to tell them more about the investigations they were about to undergo, and to those whose comments are used in this book.

Finally, many thanks to Ann Monaghan and Janet Bentham for their patience and expertise in typing and retyping the manuscript.

Figures 1–7 are reproduced, with permission, from Hubner (1980) Nurses's Guide to Cardiac Monitoring, 3rd edition, Baillière Tindall.

FOREWORD

Many patients, whether they go to their general practitioner, attend an outpatients clinic or are admitted to hospital will undergo investigations to aid in the diagnostic procedure. However simple and 'routine' these may be there is always anxiety associated with the 'unknown'.

Lack of information has been shown to increase stress, pain and may even inhibit recovery. An example of research in this area is 'Information — A Prescription Against Pain' by Jack Hayward (RCN, 1975).

These facts and the little detailed literature available on investigations led a group of third-year student nurses on the Integrated State Registration and Diploma in Nursing Course at the Middlesex Hospital to look at the problem of preparing patients for investigations, what actually happened during the investigation and the subsequent aftercare.

The original work was produced as a project and looked at the commoner investigations carried out on patients. The preparation for the final project generated a tremendous amount of interest and enthusiasm, not only among their nursing colleagues, but also amongst departmental and medical staff involved in the carrying out of investigations. This book, then, is the result of the initial project, which has been expanded to cover more of the commoner investigations normally performed. It does not set out to be a comprehensive text on all investigations. It concentrates on investigations where some preparation of the patient is required and aftercare is probable. Because of this 'routine', urine analysis and haematological tests are not included. It aims to draw people's attention to the questions which patients may actually ask or would like to ask about the investigation they are about to undergo. The questions were identified by the original work carried out for the project by the nurses.

If nurses are aware of the questions then they will be better able to prepare their patients. The book can be used by student nurses, teachers of nursing, medical students and ward staff in particular. The book may also be of use in departments where the investigations are carried out.

The format of each investigation is as follows:

1   What the investigation is.

2   Why it is being performed and what may be identified.

3   Where the investigation takes place and the preparation required which includes psychological as well as physical preparation, with particular reference to whether the investigation is likely to be painful, whether the patient will be awake and how long it is likely to last.

4   How the investigation will be carried out.

5   What will happen to the patient after the investigation is completed, including aftercare.

6   An indication as to how soon results will be known.

7   Contraindications.

8   Possible complications.

Further reading suggestions are included at the end of each chapter. In a few investigations patients' comments are included to reinforce the text.

When using the book the reader should always refer to local policy, local procedures and departmental preferences for specific details. It is impossible to include all the minor variations which occur from centre to centre.

The questions which the nurses were asked by patients which this book sets out to answer are as follows:

What is it?

What does it do?

When do I come into hospital?

What will happen before the test?

Will I be able to eat and drink?

Is there any preparation?

Will I be awake?

Will it hurt?

Do I have to do anything?

Where is it done and how do I get there?

Who will do it?

How is it done?

How long will it take?

Can complications occur?

What happens when I wake up?

What happens when I get back to the ward?

Will I be able to eat and drink afterwards?

Can I have visitors?

When will I know the results?

It should be remembered than when preparing patients one must take into account how much new information can be absorbed at any one time and medical jargon should be avoided. Explanation should be given in a way that is understandable and not confusing or frightening.

If a patient has to miss drugs, meals, fluids or other treatment this must be explained. Any possible complications resulting from this must be noted and food, fluids, drug therapy and treatment should be recommenced as soon as possible.

Even with good preparation investigations may still be frightening and tiring. When the patient returns to the ward a question about how the investigation went and how they are feeling will help the patient feel that everyone does appreciate what they have been through. The answers will also help the nurse to assess the patient's condition and so plan appropriate care.

Finally, the patient should be given the results as quickly as possible as delay will only lead to more stress and perhaps unnecessary anxiety. The ward team should decide on a policy of when and by whom the results should be given.

CHAPTER 1

INVESTIGATIONS ASSOCIATED WITH THE ALIMENTARY TRACT

The alimentary (gastrointestinal) tract is a co-ordinated system with the functions of ingesting, digesting and absorbing nutrients and excreting unabsorbed food substances and waste products.

A balanced diet is essential for normal healthy activities of growth and repair, energy and well-being of the body. It is therefore important that any malfunction of this system is diagnosed early and accurately, preferably without exploratory surgical intervention with all its associated hazards.

The following investigations are some of those which might be performed to aid diagnosis, and since they may be potentially embarrassing for the patient the nurses and other staff involved must be empathetic towards the patient.

1.1. Upper Gastrointestinal Endoscopy

What is an upper gastrointestinal endoscopy?

Upper gastrointestinal endoscopy is an investigation which allows the parts of the upper gastrointestinal tract to be visualized and, when necessary, biopsies to be taken.

What is an endoscope?   An endoscope is a fibreoptic instrument with a flexible tip down which the doctor can observe the contents, walls and movements of the upper gastrointestinal tract. Colour photographs and cine films can be taken during endoscopy and the procedure can be projected live onto a television screen and a videotape-recording taken.

Biopsy forceps can be passed through the endoscope and biopsies of selected areas and suspect lesions taken under direct vision, smears for cytological study (to see whether there are malignant cells present) can easily be obtained.

Why is an endoscopy performed?

Endoscopy may be indicated for a variety of clinical reasons and these are summarized below:

1   Dyspepsia, especially if barium X-ray is negative.
2   Dysphagia.
3   X-ray lesions, e.g., gastric ulcer.
4   Assessment of ulcer healing.
5   Preoperative assessment.
6   Symptoms after gastric surgery.
7   Iron deficiency anaemia.
8   Unexplained weight loss.
9   Unexplained vomiting.
10   Acute upper gastrointestinal bleeding.

Where is the endoscopy performed and what preparation is necessary?

The patient about to undergo routine upper gastrointestinal endoscopy is usually admitted to the ward at least one day before. The procedure can be carried out as an outpatient. The procedure should be explained to the patient by a nurse. In some hospitals where there is a gastrointestinal unit the nurse from the unit will visit the patient. The house surgeon should then visit the patient and explain the procedure again as a written consent form is needed. The patient should be fasted for at least 6 hours before the test so that there is a clear picture of the stomach. Patients with oesophageal or gastric-outlet obstruction should be fasted for longer and nasogastric aspiration may be necessary in these cases. In the morning the patient should be ready in an operation gown. False teeth, jewellery and glasses should be removed and stored somewhere safe (a note should be made of crowned teeth on the consent form). Notes, X-rays and the drugs chart should be on hand so that they can be sent down with the patient.

How is the endoscopy performed?

A silicone drink is given 5–10 min before the examination to prevent the endoscopic view being obscured by foaming. The patient should then be helped to lie comfortably in the left lateral position. The choice of local anaesthesia for the throat, analgesia and sedatives varies according to the doctor's preferences and the patient's needs, but a combination of intravenous pethidine and diazepam and benzocaine/xylocaine spray are most commonly used.

The endoscope will be passed over the tongue and down the throat into the oesophagus. The patient should not experience pain, but there may be a feeling of discomfort. Usually patients are very drowsy due to the drugs used.

What happens after the endoscopy?

The patient will be drowsy after the endoscopy and should be on bedrest until they are fully awake. He can be offered a wash and can put on his own clothes. Instructions should be sent back to the ward in the notes indicating when it is safe for the patient to eat and drink again, but if no local anaesthesia is used this is usually after 1 hour, or when awake. If an oesophageal stricture has been dilated, postinvestigational X-ray must be seen first by the doctor because of the risk of perforation of the oesophagus. There should also be instructions in the notes if any special observations are necessary, but a 4-hourly recording of temperature and pulse is usually adequate.

The patient may complain of a slight sore throat, which is normal, but any severe pain, distension or fever should be reported to the doctor. Any patients wishing to go home on the day of the investigation must be accompanied by a friend or relative and should be reminded not to drive or work for at least 24–48 hours, as they may be drowsy from the drugs.

When are the results available and what might they be?

The reports of the X-rays, pictures and any specimens taken may take a few days to come through. However, the doctor may be able to tell the patient the results within 24 hours if no biopsies were taken.

Possible findings may include:

1   Inflammation, e.g., gastritis.
2   Ulceration, e.g., chronic or acute.
3   Neoplasms, e.g., malignant or benign.
4   Anatomical abnormalities, e.g., pyloric stenosis, hiatus hernia.
5   Vascular abnormalities, e.g., oesophageal varices.

Contraindications for endoscopy

Contraindications are few, but they include severe heart disease and, especially, recent myocardial infarction. Severe respiratory disease, including active pulmonary tuberculosis, a positive blood test for Australian antigen (because this contaminates the instrument and in theory cross-infection could occur) and possible other rare conditions, such as the presence of an aortic aneurysm, are other contraindications.

Can complications occur?

The most common complication is 'over-sedation' which could lead to severe respiratory problems. Other risks include perforation of the oesophagus and stomach, chest infection through aspiration of vomit, haemorrhage and cardiac dysrhythmias. However, these complications rarely occur.

Patients' comments

'Can't remember anything! One minute I was down there and the next I was on my way back here.'

'I can only vaguely remember the tube being passed — it felt like 5 minutes, but they told me it was really an hour.'

'Well, to start with I was terrified. I can't swallow pills so I thought I'd never be able to swallow the tube. I remember the injection in my hand and talking to the nurse. Next thing I knew it was just as if someone had taken something out of my mouth. I thought it was the start, but the nurse told me it was the end. I didn't feel a thing.'

'I remember being down in the room with sister talking to me. I was very scared. I had the prick in my hand and then I was back here. It's the most marvellous thing.'

1.2.   Gastric Emptying

What are gastric emptying tests?

These are tests using isotopes and a gamma camera. The investigation determines:

1   The length of time taken for the stomach to empty.
2   The pattern of emptying.

Why are gastric emptying tests performed?

1 To confirm dumping syndrome.

2 To differentiate symptoms due to slow gastric emptying and symptoms due to dumping syndrome.

3 A research tool.

4 Prior to vagotomy — a preoperative investigation for possible fast gastric emptying.

5 Postoperatively following vagotomy, possibly with pyloroplasty, to determine effects of the surgery.

The results are available for the patient in 1–2 hours in most cases.

Where are gastric emptying tests performed and what preparation is necessary?

The investigation is usually performed in a laboratory or department away from the ward. Give the patient a full explanation of the investigation, allowing him to ask questions.

Cimetidine (Tagamet) and all drugs affecting gastric emptying are to be stopped 48 hours prior to the investigation. The patient should have nothing to eat or drink from midnight if the investigation is to be in the morning, or 8 hours prior to the test. This is to ensure the stomach is empty. The patient's notes are taken to the department with him. The patient should wear an X-ray gown and a dressing gown or be adequately covered with blankets for privacy and warmth. Jewellery should be removed and stored safely.

Feelings of nausea, fullness in the stomach, cramps, sweating and palpitations may occur. If patients are known to have dumping syndrome, they will have experienced this type of symptom after meals.

How are gastric emptying tests performed?

An intravenous cannula with a three-way tap is inserted into a vein in the arm. This enables blood samples to be taken at frequent intervals without separate venepunctures being performed. Normal saline (0.9%) can be used to flush the vein and keep it patent, though a small amount of fluid should be given as there is danger altering the patient's plasma volume. The arm must be kept still so that the cannula remains in the vein.

The patient sits in a chair and the gamma camera is positioned over the upper abdomen. The gamma camera responds to gamma-ray emission from the radioactive isotope and an image will be built up of its distribution. The camera is synchronized with a computer which stores the patient's data. A series of images of the distribution of the isotope can be reproduced on paper.

Two basal blood samples are taken from the patient, the time allowed between them is not critical. The samples are divided for two tests:

1   Haematocrit — determination of plasma volume.
2   Blood sugar levels.

When the two basal blood samples have been taken the patient drinks a mixture of radioactive isotope which emits gamma radiation — an example would be 150 ml of 50% dextrose solution labelled with 1.5 mCi of ^{113}In. The gamma camera starts recording when half the drink has been swallowed.

Blood samples are then collected from the patient every 5 min for the first 30 min, then at intervals of 40, 60, 90 and 120 min. Blood samples are again analysed for blood sugar levels and haematocrit. If the patient experiences any symptoms during the investigation they are noted. Patients who have dumping syndrome with fast gastric emptying, will experience the following:

1   Normal appetite at the start of a meal. Symptoms are precipitated by the meal and they disappear about 1 hour later.
2   Abdominal symptoms. Distension, wind, increasing discomfort, leading to possible pain, nausea, vomiting and diarrhoea.
3   Systemic symptoms. Tiredness, desire to lie down, fainting, dim vision, sweating, palpitations.

Abdominal symptoms are thought to be due to the 50% dextrose solution, which has a high osmotic pressure, drawing water from the blood towards it, therefore reducing the plasma volume. The bloated feeling is due to the extra fluid present in the small intestine.

Systemic symptoms are thought to be due to rapid absorption of carbohydrate. Insulin is secreted and all the sugars are absorbed, the stomach empties rapidly, therefore excess insulin is present in the blood, and hypoglycaemic-like symptoms are seen. It is also possible that fluid has been drawn out of the vascular compartment, reducing plasma volume, therefore hypotensive-like symptoms develop.

Patients without fast gastric emptying experience no symptoms.

A vomit bowl and tissues should be available for the patient, and a toilet should the need arise.

During the investigation an outline of the stomach can be seen on the screen, and the amount of radioactive material emptying into the duodenum is noted by the computer.

When the last blood sample has been taken, the intravenous line is removed from the patient. Patients can usually walk back to the ward, or they can be taken in a wheelchair.

The investigation takes 2 hours but only 1 hour is spent under the gamma camera.

What happens after the gastric emptying tests?

Patients tend to feel tired and possibly nauseated following this investigation, so a period of bedrest is advisable. After this a wash may be appreciated and then the patient can put on his own pyjamas. A covered vomit bowl can be placed by the bed. Symptoms normally subside after 1 hour. A normal diet and a drink of tea or coffee can be taken as soon as the patient feels like it. Prolonged nausea or vomiting should be reported to the doctor.

When are the results available and what might they be?

The results may take a few hours to come through. Possible findings include:

1   Dumping syndrome.
2   Fast emptying of the stomach.
3   Effectiveness of pyloroplasty.

Contraindications for gastric emptying tests

Patients with cardiovascular problems. Patients with diabetes can have this test performed provided the doctor is aware of this.

Can complications occur?

Complications are rare but the reproduction of dumping syndrome and loss of consciousness may occur during the test. If dumping syndrome symptoms are severe, they may cause stress to patients, therefore care and observation of frail patients is important.

1.3.   Gastric Secretion Tests (Basal and Maximal Acid Output Tests)

What are gastric secretion tests?

The acid secretion of the stomach is measured in response to the following:

1   A bolus injection of insulin to test the integrity of the vagus nerve.
2   Administration of histamine to measure gastric cell activity.
3   Pentagastrin ('test meal') to measure gastric cell activity.

Why are gastric secretion tests performed?

The reasons for doing gastric secretion tests are as follows:

1   Research into gastric physiology and pathology.
2   On patients who are suspected of having Zollinger–Ellison syndrome.
3   Postvagotomy with suspected recurrent ulcers.
4   Postvagotomy to assess effects of surgery.
5   Diagnosis of achlorhydria — pernicious anaemia.

Where are gastric secretion tests performed and what preparation is necessary?

The test is usually performed in one of the laboratories, so the patient needs to have slippers and a warm dressing gown or blanket. The patient's notes accompany him.

The tests take 4½ hours if both insulin and histamine tests are performed, therefore the patient may like to take a book or magazine to read.

The patient should be given a full explanation of the procedure, and he should be given the opportunity to ask questions. He should stop taking all anticholinergic drugs and/or cimetidine 48 hours prior to the investigation. Any antacids should also be discontinued as they will invalidate the tests.

The patient should have nothing to eat or drink from midnight if the test is in the morning, or for at least 12 hours prior to the investigation to ensure the stomach is empty. He should not smoke prior to the investigation as it may affect the results.

How is the gastric secretion test performed?

The patient's height and weight are measured before the test begins — this enables the technician to calculate the correct dose of insulin and histamine. The most uncomfortable symptoms which the patient may experience occur after the administration of the insulin, when he may have symptoms of hypoglycaemia — sweating, headache, palpitations. Some patients may react to the histamine injection — a warm flushed feeling is experienced, together with headache, dizziness and faintness.

The patient rests supine on a couch during the investigation. Some patients find it unpleasant to have the nasogastric tube inserted, so the nurse should explain to the patient exactly how it is done.

A size 14 Ryle's tube is passed into the patient's stomach via the nose. The tube is lubricated with jelly at the distal end, and the patient's throat is anaesthetized with a local anaesthetic. To aid the passage of the tube the patient is given a glass of water to drink.

When in position, the tube is secured with tape to the face and aspirated until the stomach is empty. To check the position of the tube several methods have been used — fluroscopy and the water-recovery test. In the latter test 20 ml of water is swallowed and then aspirated back. If 15–20 ml of water are recovered, the tube is pulled back 2 cm and the test repeated. When the test fails the tube is introduced again by 2 cm — the tube is then in the optimum position of the stomach.

A marker may be used, e.g., phenosulphonphthalein (PSP). This enables the doctor to detect how much gastric juice is lost through the pylorus. PSP is infused into the stomach down the nasogastric tube at a constant rate. The nasogastric tube is then continuously aspirated and gastric juice is collected at 10-min intervals for the next hour. A gastric suction pump will perform this automatically. These samples collected in the basal period are, like all the other samples, filtered and put into separate bottles. The aspirated volume is recorded each time.

During the basal period an intravenous infusion is set up with a three-way tap connected to the cannula in the patient's arm. This enables the doctor to take blood samples easily and to administer the insulin and histamine when necessary. One blood sample is collected from the patient in the basal period, and it is sent for blood glucose levels, and the cannula is flushed with 0.9% normal saline afterwards.

At the end of the hour a bolus of insulin is given intravenously — this lowers the blood sugar, the result being a stimulation of the vagus nerve which will increase gastric acid and gastrin secretion. Blood samples are then taken at 15-min intervals for the next 45 min. The gastric juice continues to be collected every 10 min for the next 2 hours.

Patients are asked to tell the doctor if they have any uncomfortable symptoms. For adequate hypoglycaemia to be achieved the blood glucose level must fall below 2.22 mmol/l. Intravenous dextrose must be at hand in case the patient goes into hypoglycaemic coma.

Following the insulin test histamine can be given, which will stimulate gastric secretion directly. Due to the side-effects of histamine, an H_1 receptor blocker (antihistamine) is given, such as Phenergan. Histamine and the H_1 receptor blocker can be given by continuous infusion or over a short period of time, depending on the response required — a plateau or peak of maximum gastric secretion. If the patient has a violent reaction to histamine then the infusion of the H_1 receptor blocker is continued, the histamine infusion is stopped.

Gastric acid samples are collected every 10 min for at least the next hour. When the test is complete the nasogastric tube is removed and the patient is offered a cup of tea or coffee. The patient is helped into a wheelchair and taken back to the ward. Outpatients are advised to have a substantial meal before undertaking a lengthy journey home, and a relative or friend should accompany them.

The gastric juice obtained can then be analysed for any of the following, depending on the policy of the hospital:

Electrolytes		*Volumes*
Hydrogen	(H^+) concentration	Total secreted volume
Chloride	(Cl^-) concentration	Pyloric loss
Sodium	(Na^+) concentration	Duodenogastric reflux
Potassium	(K^+) concentration	

The information is usually fed into a computer which produces a print-out of the results.

No increase in the production of gastric acid following the administration of histamine or pentagastrin indicates the presence of achlorhydria.

What happens after the gastric secretion tests?

When the patient returns to the ward he often feels very tired and lethargic and it is advisable to rest in bed for a short time. A normal diet and fluids can be taken by the patient as soon as he feels like it — patients are usually quite hungry.

If endoscopy is being considered, it is advisable to do this prior to gastric secretion tests as patients are left with red marks on the gastric mucosa due to the aspiration.

When are the results available and what might they be?

The results may take up to 3 days to come through. Possible findings include:

1   Recurrent ulcers.
2   Confirmation of Zollinger–Ellison Syndrome.
3   Achlorhydria.

Contraindications for gastric secretion tests

1   Patients over 60 years.
2   Epileptics.
3   Ischaemic heart disease and disabling heart conditions.
4   Diabetes — special care is required in the patient's management.
5   Sensitivity to insulin or histamine.

NOTE: Pentagastrin can also be administered subcutaneously or intramuscularly to stimulate gastric secretion. The dose is calculated according to body weight. The principles of the test are similar to those outlined for insulin and histamine. Pentagastrin does not cause the unpleasant side-effects often experienced with histamine, and the test only takes 2 hours.

Can complications occur?

Complications may include hypoglycaemia or a reaction to the histamine.

1.4.   Barium Swallow/Meal and Follow-through Examination

What is a barium swallow?

A barium meal examination is the method of investigation of the upper gastrointestinal tract using a contrast medium, so that the oesophagus, stomach and duodenum can be seen on X-ray. The procedure usually involves the introduction of gas into the stomach (from special effervescent tablets given before the examination starts) as well as the barium. This is a technique called double contrast radiography which provides a double outline so that small alterations in the gastric mucosa can be detected.

A barium swallow is a modified barium meal used when it is suspected that a lesion of the oesophagus is present. The patient is prepared as for a barium meal, but swallows a smaller amount of the barium emulsion. However, a barium swallow is not often performed on its own — it is usually performed as part of the barium meal examination.

A follow-through examination is used to demonstrate the whole of the small bowel, from the duodenojejunal flexure to the ileocaecal valve. It is a more prolonged examination in which further X-rays are taken, so the course of the barium through the intestinal tract is followed. The follow-through examination is not performed routinely as part of the barium meal/swallow, but the ward will be informed if the patient is to have this done.

Why is a barium swallow performed?

The swallow part of the examination will demonstrate lesions of the oesophagus, e.g., obstruction which may be due to a stricture, a growth or cardiospasm. If some external mass is pressing on the oesophagus, e.g., mediastinal growth or aneurysm, the course of the oesophagus will be distorted. A hiatus hernia can also be demonstrated.

By outlining the stomach, the presence of a gastric ulcer can be seen as a crater filled with barium and in early gastric cancer the mucosal folds show an altered pattern. The barium examination will also demonstrate pyloric stenosis (which may be due to an ulcer or carcinoma) leading to dilatation and a delay in emptying of the stomach. A cap appearance may indicate scar tissue of an old, healed ulcer.

The first part of the duodenal shadow forms a 'cap' which is often irregular in the case of a duodenal ulcer. If there are adhesions due to a diseased gall bladder, this may cause irregularity of the duodenal outline.

Finally, the follow-through examination is used particularly in the diagnosis of Crohn's disease, where the barium may show a narrowing of the ileum known as the 'string sign'.

Where is a barium swallow performed and what preparation is necessary?

This investigation is performed in the X-ray department. It is possible for this procedure to be carried out as an outpatient, depending on whether the patient is well enough. Usually, however, patients are admitted to hospital the day before the examination and are discharged when the results are available, unless there is a reason for them to stay. The procedure is exactly the same; the staff will ensure that the patient is fit to leave. Results are usually given at the next outpatient appointment.

NOTE: If the patient is to have the follow-through, he will need to allow the whole day for the procedure.

The patient should be given a full explanation of the procedure and should be given the opportunity to ask questions.

The patient may be quite concerned about the barium emulsion he is asked to drink, particularly if he has heard about it through other patients. The nurse can reassure the patient that it has a rather chalky taste and is slightly fizzy.

The patient should also be warned that his stools may be slightly paler in colour following the examination due to the passage of the barium.

It is essential, if the examination is to be successful, that the stomach and small bowel are empty. The preparation for a barium meal/swallow and follow-through is therefore as follows:

1 The patient must be fasted for at least 6 hours prior to the examination.

2 If the patient is to have a follow-through examination he should have an aperient on the two nights preceding the examination and check that the bowel is empty.

3 Immediately before the examination the patient should don an X-ray gown and remove any necklaces or jewellery.

4 Before leaving the ward the patient should empty his bladder.

How is a barium swallow performed?

When the patient arrives in the X-ray department he will be asked to take some effervescent tablets which react with the acid in the stomach causing a release of gas which provides the double contrast. Sometimes an antispasmodic agent is given intramuscularly to reduce spasm in the gastrointestinal tract. The patient is then asked to stand on the foot rest of the X-ray table, which is in the vertical position behind the screen.

During the swallow part of the examination the patient is asked to hold the barium in his mouth and swallow it at a precise moment as directed by the radiologist. This is so that an X-ray can be taken of the barium lining the whole of the oesophagus. The patient then drinks the barium emulsion (about 200–300 ml) while its passage down the oesophagus, into the stomach and duodenum is observed on a monitor.

X-rays are taken at intervals and in different positions, both standing upright and lying down. The latter is achieved by tilting the X-ray table into a horizontal position.

A barium swallow/meal usually takes 20–30 min, but it may take much longer if the patient is having a follow-through examination. If the patient is having the follow-through, he will be asked to lie down in a waiting room in the X-ray department after the barium meal, and X-rays are taken at $\frac{1}{2}$-hourly intervals. The patient remains in the department until the examination is finished, so he may wish to take a book with him.

The barium meal and follow-through will certainly take up the whole morning and may continue throughout the afternoon. An injection of metaclopramide may be given to speed the movement of barium through the tract. Results are usually available within 1–3 days of the examination once the medical team have had time to study the X-rays.

What happens after a barium swallow?

There is no specific aftercare following a barium meal or follow-through. However, it can be a tiring procedure, so the patient may wish to lie down and rest for a short while on return to the ward.

The patient can eat and drink normally afterwards and should be encouraged to do so as this will help relieve any nausea he might have or feeling of indigestion, and it will also encourage the passage of the barium.

When are the results available and what might they be?

The results are available within 1–3 days, and might include

1   Obstruction, due to a growth, stricture or cardiospasm.
2   Hiatus hernia.
3   Gastric ulcer.
4   Pyloric stenosis.
5   Duodenal ulcer.
6   Crohn's disease.

Contraindications

This procedure should not be performed on a person where there is a risk of perforation, e.g., a patient with bleeding gastric ulcer or someone with intestinal obstruction.

Diabetic patients — the X-ray department should be notified if the patient has diabetes mellitus, so that he can be given the earliest appointment of the day. If taking insulin or other agents, the patient should miss his breakfast, but arrangements must be made for him to have his normal meal as soon as the examination is completed. If he is on insulin or other diabetic agents, he should omit the morning dose as well as breakfast, but again arrangements must be made for these to be available at the earliest opportunity.

Can complications occur?

The main complication associated with any investigation of the gastrointestinal tract using barium is constipation. Rarely, it may cause obstruction. Therefore, if the patient does not have his bowels open within 3 days it may be necessary to intervene and give an aperient or enemata. However, the patient's normal bowel habit should be taken into account before any action is taken.

Patients' comments

'I had nothing to eat for a few hours. Went down to the X-ray room. Did feel a little nervous. I was told to drink some crystal stuff, which was junk liquid and tasted horrible. It made my mouth feel sticky. Had to drink water as well. X-rays were taken as I drank and it was all over in 10 min.'

'Not so bad really. Worst thing was not being able to have my breakfast before the investigation because you can't eat or drink for some time before. I had to drink some strange mixture, but it was all right. It didn't make me feel sick at all.'

'I had to drink quite a lot of water with a strange solution. Tasted rather nasty, but I didn't mind because it was necessary for the doctor to get a very good picture of my insides. Very clever because the doctor was able to look at the X-ray pictures and tell me what he could see. Very quick and easy. Nothing to worry about.'

1.5. Barium Enema

What is a barium enema?

A barium enema examination is the method of investigation of the colon by retrograde injection of a contrast medium so that the colon can be seen on X-ray. The procedure usually involves the use of radio-opaque and radiotranslucent contrast media, e.g., barium sulphate and air, thus producing a double contrast. This enables small mucosal lesions, e.g., polyps, to be detected which might otherwise be missed.

Why is a barium enema performed?

A barium enema is a diagnostic tool for identifying abnormalities of the colon. It will demonstrate obstruction due to malignant growths; the presence of diverticular disease and strictures; and show up small mucosal lesions, e.g., polyps. In ulcerative colitis the outline of the bowel has fine irregularities and will show loss of haustration.

Where is a barium enema performed and what preparation is necessary?

The examination takes place in the X-ray department. It is possible to have a barium enema examination performed as an outpatient, depending on whether the patient is well enough. Usually patients are admitted 1 or 2 days prior to the examination and discharged once the results are available, unless there is a reason why they need to stay.

The procedure is exactly the same for an outpatient, except that he will be given the castor oil to take at home and the veripaque enema and high colonic washout will be performed in the X-ray department. The patient will need to allow the whole morning for the examination and will probably not feel like returning to work. The X-ray staff will ensure that he is well enough to leave, and the results will be given at the next outpatient visit or sent to the general practitioner.

The patient should be given a full explanation of the procedure and also be given a chance to ask questions. This should reduce anxiety, which is known to cause the procedure to be painful. The patient can be told that a barium enema is not usually painful, but it is often uncomfortable and is accompanied by a sensation of fullness in the gut. If haemorrhoids are present then some degree of pain may be experienced. The patient should also be warned that following the examination his stools may become pale in colour due to the passage of the barium.

The colon must be cleared of faecal material before the examination can be successful. The preparation for a barium enema is as follows:

1 During the 2 days preceding the examination the patient should have a low residue diet, e.g., cheese, eggs, fish, white bread and butter. He should avoid meat, vegetables and fruit in any form.

2 The patient is given 30 ml castor oil at midday on the day before the examination.

3 On the day of the examination the patient is allowed fluids only and should *not* eat anything.

4 A veripaque enema followed by a high colonic washout (see hospital procedure book) should be performed on the morning of the examination, not the night before.

5 The patient should undress completely and don a hospital gown.

NOTE: It is important that the preparation be carried out properly as poor preparation may mean a repeat of the examination.

How is a barium enema performed?

The patient is asked to lie on the table in the left lateral position, with the knees drawn up. Privacy and dignity will be maintained. Once the patient is comfortable a rectal tube (to which a bag containing barium sulphate is attached) is inserted into the rectum. This may feel uncomfortable, but not painful. The barium sulphate is slowly run into the bowel while being observed on a monitor. The patient is asked to adopt different positions during the procedure — in particular, he is asked to turn from his left side onto his right so that the barium coats the whole of the large bowel.

The barium is then run out of the bowel via the rectal tube and air is pumped into the bowel to provide a double contrast, and to separate the mucosal folds. X-rays are taken and the table may be tipped at this stage into the vertical position, so that the patient is standing upright, being supported by the foot rest at the end of the table.

Once all the necessary pictures have been taken and the rectal tube is removed, the patient is allowed to go to the toilet to evacuate the barium and air left in the bowel.

The procedure usually takes about ½ hour.

What happens after a barium enema?

There is no specific postinvestigative care. However, it is sometimes overlooked that the investigation can be an uncomfortable and embarrassing one for the patient, and it may be quite an ordeal for the elderly or frail person. The patient will therefore need time to lie down and rest following a barium enema.

The patient may eat or drink normally on return to the ward.

When are the results available and what might they be?

The results are usually available in 1–3 days when the medical team have had time to study the X-rays. Possible results include obstruction due to malignant growth; diverticular disease and strictures; polyps.

Contraindications for a barium enema

A barium enema should not be performed on a person where there is a risk of perforation of the bowel, or where there is known to be a fistula.

Can complications occur?

The main complication following a barium enema examination is constipation, so that if the patient does not have his bowels open within 3 days of the examination it may be necessary to intervene and give an aperient or enema. However, the patient's normal bowel habits should be considered first.

Occasionally, while the barium is being run into the bowel, the patient suffers cramp-like pain due to spasm of the colon. This may be relieved by the intramuscular administration of an antispasmodic agent.

Patients' comments

'Had to have a big enema the night before. This was rather unpleasant, but it was to clear me out so that the investigation would be good. I had nothing to eat on the day and went down to the X-ray department. I did feel shaky and nervous. I was made to lay on the table on my left side facing the X-ray machines. I was given an enema and they told me to let them know if it was uncomfortable. I was able to stand it for 8 min. It wasn't painful at all, but a tiny bit uncomfortable. It isn't really too bad.'
'They put some enema fluid into me and took pictures to see the fluid in my body. It meant that the doctor could see my inside without doing an operation. It was good and over very quickly.'
'I couldn't feel the fluid as it went in, but I did feel a little uncomfortable. Afterwards when I went to the toilet I passed some white motion, but this is very normal I was told.'

1.6.   Collection of Faecal Specimens for Occult Blood

What is an occult blood test?

Occult means 'hidden'. Occult blood, therefore, is blood which has passed into the alimentary tract, usually in small amounts, and during the passage along the tract becomes mixed with the faeces and altered by the digestive juices so that it is not obvious to the naked eye. It can only be detected by chemical tests.

Why is an occult blood test performed?

The occult blood test is an additional factor in the diagnosis of gastric and duodenal ulcers and can give a guide as to whether they have healed or not. Occult blood will be positive in an active ulcer and negative in a healed ulcer. It is continuously positive in cases of carcinoma of the stomach or growths in any other part of the alimentary tract. If there is a lot of altered blood present the stools may look black — melaena stools.
NOTE: Iron, bismuth and manganese also cause stools to look black.

What preparation is necessary?

The patient should ideally abstain from eating red meat 3 days prior to collecting the specimen as substances present in these foods may occasionally invalidate the result.

Drugs like asprin should be stopped 3 days prior to the collection because of the irritant effect on the gastric mucosa.

How is a faecal specimen collected?

The patient is asked to use a bedpan the next time he has his bowels open. A small quantity of faeces is put into a wax cardboard carton or specimen pot, labelled and sent to the laboratory.

How is an occult blood test performed?

The presence of blood is detected by placing a small bead of faeces on a test paper and a tablet placed on top. The reagent or dilutent is placed on top of the tablet and colour changes are observed. The most common reagents used are Okokit, Peronome or Hemofec. The result is either positive or negative.

When are the results available and what might they be?

The results will be available in 2–3 days. Possible findings may be positive in an active ulcer and negative in a healed ulcer. Occult blood is continuously positive in cases of carcinoma of the stomach or growths in other parts of the alimentary tract.

1.7.   Endoscopic Retrograde Cholangio Pancreatography (ERCP)

What is endoscopic retrograde cholangio pancreatography (ERCP)?

ERCP is the procedure whereby a side-viewing fibreoptic endoscope is passed to the second part of the duodenum and from there a fine catheter is passed through the instrument and introduced into the ampulla of Vater. This enables a contrast medium to be injected into the pancreatic duct and biliary tree and any abnormalities should show up under X-ray screening. Biopsy and cytology specimens may also be taken.

Why is an ERCP performed?

It is used to aid differential diagnosis of the following:

1 Pancreatic duct obstruction or distortion caused by chronic pancreatitis or pancreatic carcinoma.

2 Obstructive jaundice.

3 Cause of high abdominal pain following ingestion of fatty foods.

4 Biliary stones, which can then be removed.

Where is an ERCP performed and what preparation is necessary?

The preparation is very similar to that of the patient about to have an upper gastrointestinal endoscopy (see Section 1.1). The patient is admitted to the ward, usually a couple of days before the procedure, as the doctor may wish to carry out certain pancreatic function tests (see Section 3.2), or have an ultrasound report first (see Section 9.2).

The procedure should be explained to the patient by a nurse the day before the ERCP and the patient should be given a chance to ask questions. In some hospitals where there is a gastrointestinal unit the nurse from the unit will visit the patient. The house-officer should then visit the patient and explain the procedure again as a written consent is needed. He will also take blood for coagulation studies, grouping and cross-matching.

The patient should be fasted for at least 8 hours prior to the test so that there is a clear picture of the stomach and duodenum in order for the ampulla of Vater to be cannulated. Immediately before the procedure the patient needs to be ready in an operation gown — pyjama trousers should not be worn as the diathermy pad is attached to the patient's thigh. False teeth, jewellery and glasses should be removed and stored somewhere safe. Notes, X-rays and the drug chart should be on hand so that they can be sent down with the patient.

How is an ERCP performed?

A silicone drink is given to the patient 5–10 min before the examination to prevent the endoscopic view being obscured by foaming. The patient should then be helped to lie comfortably in the left lateral position. He is usually turned fully prone when the endoscope has entered the second part of the duodenum, so this initial positioning makes it easier to move him when he is sedated. If diathermy is likely to be used the plate is strapped to the patient's thigh at this stage.

The choice of analgesia, sedatives and local anaesthetic for the throat varies according to the doctor's preference and the patient's needs, but a combination of intravenous pethidine and diazepam and benzocaine/xylocaine spray are most commonly used. The mouthguard is then put into position and the lubricated endoscope is passed over the tongue and the patient is asked to swallow so that the endoscope passes down the oesophagus. The patient should not experience pain and discomfort is minimal if the patient is well sedated.

Buscopan (hyoscine butylbromide) is given to suppress the duodenal motor activity so that the fine catheter can pass into the ampulla of Vater. The contrast medium is then slowly injected under X-ray screening control and the duct systems identified. X-ray films are taken during the procedure.

If a stone or stones are seen in the common bile duct the doctor may perform a sphincterotomy. This means that a diathermy wire is inserted through the biopsy channel of the endoscope and the sphincter of Oddi cut to allow the stones to pass. The stones are sometimes removed after sphincterotomy using a basket or balloon catheter. Occasionally a fine plastic tube may be left in the bile duct and re-routed from the mouth to the nose. This nasobiliary tube may be left in place for several days and does not interfere with eating and drinking. The tube allows the injection of contrast medium for cholangiography after 24–48 hours to check that all duct stones have passed. If they have not passed the tube may be used to flush the duct with a dextrose/saline solution. If this fails, a repeat ERCP may be necessary after a few days and basket extraction attempted again.

What happens after an ERCP?

The patient will be drowsy after the ERCP and should remain in bed until he is fully awake. A wash should be offered and his own night clothes can be put on. Instructions should be sent back in the notes indicating when it is safe for the patient to eat and drink again, but this is usually when he is fully awake. If a local anaesthetic has been applied to the throat the patient should be fasted for at least 1 hour to allow it time to wear off. If a sphincterotomy has been performed the patient is commonly starved for at least 4 hours, or until seen by the doctor, as an empty stomach is important because of the risk of bleeding. There should also be instructions in the notes if any special observations are necessary. After complex ERCP examinations it is necessary to record 4-hourly observations of temperature, pulse and blood pressure for 24 hours. After a sphincterotomy ½-hourly recordings of pulse and blood pressure are taken for at least the first 4 hours because of the risk of haemorrhage.

The patient may complain of a slight sore throat, which is normal, but any severe pain, distension or fever should be reported to the doctor.

When are the results available and what might they be?

The doctor will usually tell the patient the results within 24 hours. However, if biopsies have been taken it will take a few days before the results are known. Possible findings could include:

1   Stone in common bile duct.

2   Carcinoma of the head of the pancreas.

3   Pancreatitis with scarring and fibrosis.

4   Benign stricture of the common bile duct following surgery.

Contraindications for an ERCP

Contraindications are very few, but they include severe heart disease, especially recent myocardial infarction, severe respiratory disease, including active pulmonary tuberculosis, a positive blood test for Australian antigen (because this contaminates the instrument and in theory cross-infection could occur) and possibly other rare situations such as the presence of an aortic aneurysm.

Can complications occur?

ERCP carries the same, but rare, risks as upper gastrointestinal endoscopy, i.e., sore throat, venous thrombosis, respiratory depression due to oversedation or inhalation of secretions and shock due to perforation or bleeding. In addition:

1   The use of large doses of Buscopan may give rise to blurred vision or retention of urine.

2 The injection of contrast medium into the biliary and pancreatic ducts may provoke infection (cholangitis) and pancreatitis.

3 After sphincterotomy there is a risk of acute bleeding (haematemesis or melaena) during the first 24 hours.

Patients' comments

'I can't remember a thing. I remember being taken down to X-ray and talking to the nurse there and then being back here.'

'I was very frightened when I heard I wouldn't be unconscious when they put the tube down. I can't swallow tablets well so I never thought I would be able to swallow this tube, but to be honest I didn't feel a thing.'

'I had seen the programme about this test on the television so I knew what to expect, and with everyone explaining so clearly what was going to happen I shouldn't have been worried, but really I still was terrified. It's the thought of swallowing that tube. Anyhow, it happened very quickly, or so it seemed, and I didn't feel a thing.'

1.8.   Sigmoidoscopy

What is a sigmoidoscopy?

Sigmoidoscopy is an investigation which allows the upper rectum, rectosigmoid junction and lower pelvic colon to be visualized and, when necessary, biopsies to be taken.

What is a sigmoidoscope?

The sigmoidoscope is a hollow, fibreoptic tube about 30 cm long. Through this it is possible to see the mucosa and any presenting abnormalities, such as an excess of mucus, the presence of blood, ulceration, neoplasm or disease of the mucosa. Biopsies of the mucosa or lesions can be taken and provide important diagnostic information.

Why is sigmoidoscopy performed?

It is used to aid differential diagnosis of the following:

1 Polyps.

2 Carcinoma of the rectum.

3   Ulcerative colitis.

4   Crohn's disease.

5   Diverticulitis.

Where is the sigmoidoscopy performed and what preparation is necessary?

This investigation can be carried out in the outpatient clinic, in a hospital in the ward, in a special gastroenterology department, or by a general practitioner who has undertaken special training. Instructions will be sent to the patient.

A full simple explanation is needed before the examination to help ensure patient cooperation. The patient also needs to be forewarned of the small degree of discomfort which accompanies the procedure. Some patients experience pain if they are very anxious or if haemorrhoids are present.

The advance preparation of the patient for sigmoidoscopy tends to be variable. If the doctor plans the investigation in advance, a small phosphate enema may be given the night before. In an emergency, it is performed with no preparation. It is always advisable to check with the doctor carrying out the investigation.

How is sigmoidoscopy performed?

The patient should be positioned in the left lateral position with the knees drawn up to the chest and the buttocks just over the side of the bed. This ensures a clear view of the sigmoid colon. An incontinence pad should be placed beneath the buttocks. A blanket to cover the patient helps to reduce any embarrassment, and should ensure minimal exposure. Complete privacy and a warm environment are also essential. The presence of a nurse is a great reassurance to the patient. The patient should also be forewarned that air will be pumped into the bowel during the procedure to improve the view of the mucosa. This may produce a feeling of distension which may cause the patient to think that he is about to open his bowels. In fact, faecal incontinence during a sigmoidoscopy is rare. The passing of flatus should also be blamed on the air and the patient's embarrassment relieved. The discrete use of 'fresh air' spray or Airwick may be useful.

The instruments should be warm and well lubricated before they are used to minimize discomfort. When the instrument is in position, the air will be pumped into the bowel, so that a clear field of vision is obtained.

If any biopsies are taken these should be placed in specimen pots, clearly labelled and sent immediately to the pathology department.

What happens after the sigmoidoscopy?

The patient should be made comfortable after the investigation. After a rest, he is usually able to get up. If a biopsy has been taken the patient should be warned that a small quantity of blood may be visible in the next motion passed, and that this need not be a cause for concern. More profuse bleeding following a rectal biopsy is not unknown, but is extremely rare.

When are the results available and what might they be?

Any histological reports should be available within 3–4 days. Possible findings include:

1   Polyps.
2   Carcinoma of the rectum.
3   Ulcerative colitis.
4   Crohn's disease.
5   Diverticulitis.

Contraindications for sigmoidoscopy.

There are no contraindications.

Can complications occur?

Complications are rare, but perforation of the colon could occur, also profuse haemorrhage following a biopsy. Discomfort may be experienced, but acute pain is not commonly felt.

1.9.   Liver Biopsy

What is a liver biopsy?

A liver biopsy is where a small piece of liver tissue is removed with a small puncture needle. It is sometimes called a 'needle biopsy'.

Why is a liver biopsy performed?

A liver biopsy enables liver tissue to be obtained for histological examination without the dangers of general anaesthesia. From this many conditions can be diagnosed including cirrhosis of the liver, neoplasms, amyloidosis and miliary tuberculosis.

Where is the liver biopsy performed and what preparation is necessary?

Liver biopsy is performed in the ward. Before the biopsy is taken bleeding, clotting, prothrombin times and platelet counts must be taken in order to exclude any bleeding tendency. If the prothrombin time is prolonged an injection of vitamin K may be given. The patient's blood must also be grouped and cross-matched so that it is available if haemorrhage occurs. Liver function tests should also be carried out (see Section 1.10). A full and simple explanation of the procedure should be given to the patient to help ensure patient cooperation, and the patient's questions should be answered.

How is the liver biopsy performed?

Half an hour before the test a mild tranquillizer, such as diazepam (Valium), may be given. A sterile trolley is prepared as per hospital procedure. Privacy and dignity are maintained. The patient is positioned lying on his back with one pillow; he will have his right hand under his head and his right side parallel to the edge of the bed. He must be able to follow the doctor's breathing instructions precisely during the procedure.

The skin over and around the liver is cleaned with sterile swabs. Local anaesthetic is then injected to the appropriate area. When this has taken effect the biopsy is performed using a special puncture needle to remove a small portion of liver tissue. Local pressure will be experienced by the patient. The tissue is then placed in a specimen pot, labelled and sent to the laboratory for histology.

What happens after the liver biopsy?

The puncture site is dressed (occlusive dressing or air strip dressing may be used — it can be removed after 48 hours). The patient is made comfortable. He should remain on bedrest for 24 hours. For the first hour he should lie on the right side to give some direct pressure on the biopsy site. Observations of pulse and blood pressure are recorded every $\frac{1}{4}$ hour for 2 hours, and then hourly for the next 22 hours. By doing this any signs of internal haemorrhage will be quickly noticed. The puncture site should also be inspected.

A wash may be appreciated and the patient can put his own night clothes on. The patient can eat and drink as soon as he feels he wants to.

When are the results available and what might they be?

The results from the laboratory may take a few days to come through before the doctor can inform the patient. Possible findings include:

1   Cirrhosis of the liver.

2   Neoplasms.

3   Amyloidosis.

4   Miliary tuberculosis.

Contraindications for a liver biopsy.

There are no contraindications.

Can complications occur?

These are very rare. If full aspesis is maintained, infection is unlikely. Haemorrhage could occur, but close observation of the patient should detect this.

Patients' comments

'I felt more anticipation than fear, but can honestly say that it is nothing that needs to be worried about — nothing to write home about.'

'The doctor anaesthetized an area of my right side towards the back. Then a needle was put into my side. It only lasted about 5 min. I felt a feeling of discomfort, but no pain.'

'I felt a bit of soreness on my side, but nothing to shout about!'

1.10.   Liver Function Tests

What are liver function tests?

The liver, one of the largest and most vascular organs of the body, is also multifunctional. Disease, drugs or trauma which interfere with any of its many functions will quickly disturb normal homoeostasis and the functions of the rest of the body.

Most of the major functions of the liver can be studied by tests of blood, urine or stools. Liver function tests include studies of the liver's ability to metabolize bilirubin, carbohydrates, proteins and fats.

Why are liver function tests performed?

1   To aid in differential diagnosis of jaundice.

2   To confirm suspected liver disease.

3   To estimate liver function as a guide to progress and an aid to prognosis.

Where are liver function tests performed and what preparation is necessary?

Most of the blood tests will take place in the ward. No preparation is required for most of the blood tests.

How is the liver function test performed?

The tests will involve the doctor taking a blood sample from the patient's arm. He will put a tight rubber cuff around the upper arm and will ask the patient to clench and unclench his fist several times to make a vessel more accessible. The doctor will then clean the area where he is going to take the sample with an antiseptic or spirit, which will feel cold. He will insert a needle into the vessel and withdraw blood into a syringe. The cuff is then released. The prick will be felt, but the rest of the procedure should be pain-free. Once the specimen has been taken the needle will be withdrawn and a swab will be put over the injection site.

Some of the tests are:

1   **Estimation of serum bilirubin**   The normal total bilirubin values are 3–17 mmol/l. This test is valuable in diagnosing jaundice and assessing its severity.

2   **The serum protein**   Some of the most important functions of the liver are concerned with protein metabolism, including amino acids and maintenance of normal levels of albumin, globulin and fibrinogen in the blood. Determination of the ratio of serum proteins to A/G ratio is a measure of hepatic function. The ratio is 1.2:2.4. Total albumin 35–50 g/l, total globulin 20–33 g/l. An alteration in the normal ratio may indicate degenerative disease of the liver. No fasting is required for this test.

3   **Prothrombin levels**   Prothrombin levels are often lowered in biliary

obstruction, cirrhosis of the liver, metastatic carcinoma of the liver and acute hepatic necrosis.

4   **Excretory Function (BSP test)**   The liver is an organ of excretion and by giving a dye, Bromosulphthalein (BSP), the excretion of the dye can be monitored and it gives an indication of liver cell function and of the circulation to the liver.

What preparation will be needed for this test?

The patient is weighed so that the dosage of dye can be given accordingly (5 mg/kg body weight). Patients are fasted for 6 hours prior to the test.

How long will the test last?

About 1 hour.

How will the test be carried out?

An injection of Bromosulphthalein is injected into the forearm vein. This is done slowly because of the risk of anaphylactic reaction. Thirty minutes later a specimen of blood will be taken from the opposite forearm and hepatic BSP uptake is deduced from the amount retained in the serum. High levels of retention, greater than 10% is abnormal.

What happens after the liver function test?

The doctor will ask the patient to apply pressure over the site where the blood was taken from for 2 min. After this time, if no further leakage occurs, the swab can be disposed of.

When are the results available?

The doctor will send the blood to the laboratory and after examination the results will be available for the ward doctor in 2–3 days.

Contraindications for liver function tests

Phenolphthalein tests for kidney function should not be scheduled for at least 24 hours after the dye has been given.

Can complications occur?

Anaphylactic shock might occur if the patient is allergic to the injection.

1.11.   Abdominal Paracentesis

What is abdominal paracentesis?

Abdominal paracentesis is the puncturing of the abdominal wall to withdraw fluid, known as ascites, from the peritoneal cavity.

The peritoneal cavity contains serous fluid which acts as a lubricant and allows the abdominal organs to move smoothly over one another. The overproduction of fluid causing ascites gives rise to a progressive distension of the abdomen causing pressure on other structures such as the diaphragm, and the patient may complain of dyspnoea.

Why is abdominal paracentesis performed?

Abdominal paracentesis is carried out to relieve the symptoms caused by the pressure and also to find the underlying cause for the overproduction of the fluid.

Ascites can be due to:

1   Heart failure.
2   Peritonitis.
3   Carcinoma or tuberculosis of the peritoneum.
4   Renal failure.
5   Liver disease.
6   Obstruction of the portal vein.

The ascitic fluid may be:

1   Clear.
2   Turbid when due to infection.
3   Blood stained when due to abdominal malignancy.

Where is abdominal paracentesis performed and what preparation is necessary?

Abdominal paracentesis should be carefully explained to the patient as the doctor may require some co-operation during the procedure. Immediately beforehand the bladder should be voided; catheterization may be indicated. This is important as there is a danger of piercing the wall of the bladder. The abdominal site may require shaving if the patient is hirsute.

The patient should be positioned sitting upright supported with pillows.

Patients with gross ascites experience great discomfort. Therefore, care must be taken when moving and positioning the patient to achieve comfort and maximum drainage. An abdominal binder may be placed in position so that it can be applied as soon as the paracentesis is performed, pressure being required from the upper abdomen downwards.

How is abdominal paracentesis performed?

This is an aseptic procedure performed by a doctor. The nurse will be required to help with opening sterile packs, but her first responsibility is to care for the patient.

A trolley should be prepared as for an aseptic technique with the equipment required. The patient's bladder should be empty, then the patient should be screened and positioned, sitting upright and supported by pillows. Privacy and dignity must be maintained. The trolley should be conveniently positioned for the doctor who should then organize the sterile field and apparatus. The nurse should check the local anaesthetic with the doctor and open and hold the ampoule so that the doctor can draw it up. A small amount of local anaesthetic is then injected into the site chosen for insertion of the trochar and cannula. The patient may feel the initial prick and slight burning sensation as the local anaesthetic is injected.

A small incision is made, after which the cannula is inserted. (A small gauze dressing may be applied and the cannula fixed with strapping — check that the patient is not allergic to the strapping.) Silicone tubing is attached to the cannula and the other end attached to a drainage bag. The tubing has a regulating attachment.

The rate of drainage should be regulated by the doctor and controlled by the regulating attachment on the tubing by the nurse. Usually the rate is 1–2 l over 24 hours, although larger amounts can be drained in patients with gross ascites. There is a risk of shock in patients losing a large quantity of fluid too quickly, therefore regular recording of the pulse rate should be made to monitor the patient's condition and for early detection of shock.

A specimen of withdrawn fluid should be sent to the laboratories for investigations into the cause of the ascites.

What happens after abdominal paracentesis?

The cannula remains in position for as long as drainage occurs. If applied, the abdominal binder needs to be tightened as the ascites decrease. Daily care of the cannula site is important to prevent infection. Once fluid has drained (often over a period of days) the cannula should be removed and a suitable occlusive dressing applied to the wound, as some leakage may occur.

NOTE: If drainage stops, a change in position may promote further drainage.

The cannula will be removed using a strict aseptic technique on doctor's instructions, when drainage has ceased. This should not be painful. The site should have an occlusive dressing applied. It should be inspected for leakage. Healing will occur within a few days dependent on the patient's condition.

The patient should be observed for signs of shock, including pulse, blood pressure, general colour and condition, discomfort or pain. The wound site should be observed and the dressing removed once the wound is clean and dry.

The patient should sit well up to encourage drainage, but may need to be nursed from side to side to relieve pressure areas. A bed cradle may help to relieve pressure on the cannula. Full nursing care is apropriate if the patient is very ill, and great care must be taken when lifting and positioning. As the ascites reduce the patient should feel more comfortable and dyspnoea should reduce.

Contraindications for abdominal paracentesis

There are no contraindications.

Can complications occur?

Complications may include shock, infection of the wound site peritonitis and perforation of the bladder wall.

Patients' comments

'I call it my "draining out". Before I had this procedure I had fluid and water in my middle. The doctor put an anaesthetic into my tummy and then inserted a needle. I felt the needle go in — a strange sensation — but it did not hurt. The doctor then let some fluid drain away from out of the needle into a bag. This did not hurt at all. I remember the fluid was warm. It was nothing to be frightened about and the doctor explained everything exactly.'

Further Reading

Armstrong P and Wastie M (1981) X-Ray Diagnosis, Blackwell Scientific

Baron J (1979) Clinical Tests of Gastric Secretion — History, Methods and Interpretation, OUP

Bateson M and Bouchier I (1981) Clinical Investigations of Gastrointestinal Function, 2nd edition, Blackwell Scientific

Beck M (1981) Diagnostic tests: intestinal tests, Nursing (US) 11: 20–24

Beck M (1981) Diagnostic tests: common gastrointestinal tests and how to help your patient through each, Nursing (US) 11: 34–35

Chesney D and Chesney M (1978) Care of the Patient in Diagnostic Radiography, Blackwell Scientific

Clarke M (1977) Practical Nursing, Baillière Tindall

Cotton P and Williams B (1980) Practical Gastrointestinal Endoscopy, Blackwell Scientific

Gary C and Howarth P (1981) Clinical Chemical Pathology, 9th edition, Edward Arnold

Gillespie I and Thomson J (1977) Gastroenterology, 2nd edition, Churchill Livingstone

Gibson J (1979) Modern Medicine for Nurses, 4th edition, Blackwell Scientific

Hadfield J and Hobsley M (1978) Current Surgical Practice, Volume 2, Problems after Gastric Surgery, Edward Arnold

Hollander D (1979) Gastrointestinal Endoscopy, Baillière Tindall

Luckmann J and Sorenson K (1980) Medical–Surgical Nursing, 2nd edition, Saunders

MacLeod J (editor) (1981) Davidson's Principles and Practice of Medicine, 13th edition, Churchill Livingstone

Petlin A (1982) Getting your patient through lower gastrointestinal bleeding, Registered Nurse 45: 42–47

Rice A (1978) Gastrointestinal Nursing, Medical Examination Publishing

Royal College of Nursing (1981) A Guide to Endoscopy Nursing, Rcn

Shafer K (1980) Medical–Surgical Nursing, 7th edition, Mosby

Sheiner H (1975) Gastric emptying tests in man, Gut 16: 235–247

Smalley J (1976) Bowel Preparation in Abdominal Radiology, Norgine

Sykes M (1981) Aspects of Gastroenterology for Nurses, Pitman Medical

Truelove S and Reynell P (1972) Diseases of the Digestive System, 2nd edition, Blackwell Scientific

Vellacott K and Hardcastle J (1981) Evaluation of flexible fibreoptic sigmoidoscopy, British Medical Journal 283: 1583–1586

Weir J and Abrahams P (1978) Atlas of Radiological Anatomy, Pitman Medical

CHAPTER 2

INVESTIGATIONS ASSOCIATED WITH THE CARDIOVASCULAR AND LYMPHATIC SYSTEMS

The cardiovascular system, comprising of the heart and arterial system, is responsible for providing an adequate blood supply, containing the necessary nutrients and oxygen for normal activity, to the tissues. The veins carry blood, rich in nutrients and waste products of metabolism, and associated lymphatic vessels carry lymph, which comprises of tissue fluid, particulate matter and dissolved substances, back to the heart and eventually to the kidneys where excretion of the waste products of metabolism and excess water can take place.

Disease, damage or drugs which interfere with effective cardiac activity will, therefore, interfere with normal body function. Interference with the flow of blood or lymph in the vessels will lead to alteration of the delicate distribution of fluid around the body. Investigations associated with the heart, blood or lymphatic system can cause alarm and so clear explanations must always be given. Complications can occur so patients and relatives must be prepared. Careful monitoring of the patient's condition postinvestigation will in many cases ensure that complications will be identified if they develop and appropriate action taken.

2.1. Electrocardiogram (ECG)

What is an ECG?

The electrocardiogram records the electrical charges associated with cardiac contractions and these are represented in the form of a graphic chart or displayed on an ECG monitor. The spread of the heartbeat is initiated from the sino-atrial node (S-A node) situated in the right atrium, close to the entry of the superior vena cava. From here the heartbeat spreads out through the atrial muscle and brings about contraction of both the atria. This action is represented by the P wave. Depolarization then spreads through the atrio-ventricular node, also in the right atrium. Between the atria and ventricles there is a fibrous septum in which is situated the Bundle of His, which is a conduction pathway to the ventricles. The Bundle of His branches into the Purkinje fibres thus allowing electrical depolarization to spread rapidly through the muscle mass and ventricular contraction follows. This is represented on the ECG graph as the QRS complex. The T wave represents repolarization, which occurs in diastole (Figure 1). The duration of the waves and complexes of the electrocardiogram varies from beat to beat and from person to person. However, the normal durations are:

PR segment = 0.12–0.21 seconds.
QRS complex = 0.08–0.11 seconds.

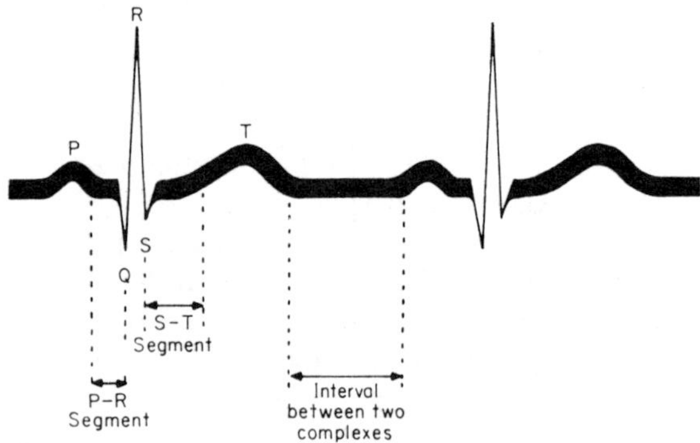

Figure 1.   Normal ECG trace. P Wave + QRS complex + T Wave = one complex. QRS complex + T wave = one QRS–T complex.

Why is an ECG performed?

An ECG is performed

1   As a routine investigation prior to surgery to ensure that there are no cardiac problems or abnormalities which could become serious during surgery.

2   To establish a baseline status of cardiac function.

3   Following myocardial infarction and coronary thrombosis to assess the extent of damage.

4   To show the stage of heartblock and the presence of ectopic beats (a heartbeat originating from another part of the heart other than the S-A node).

Cardiac monitoring is used routinely in the intensive care units and coronary care units to monitor closely the conditions of the patients' hearts.

Possible results and findings could include the following:

1   Myocardial infarction.

2   Ischaemic heart disease.

In these conditions the ventricle has an insufficient blood supply from the coronary arteries and one ventricle does not produce its full voltage. This will be seen on the ECG in the part called the S–T segment. The direction of displacement of the S–T segment will enable the site of the thrombosis to be determined. With an anterior thrombosis there is a raised S–T segment (Figure 2) and with a posterior thrombosis there is a depressed S–T segment (Figure 3).

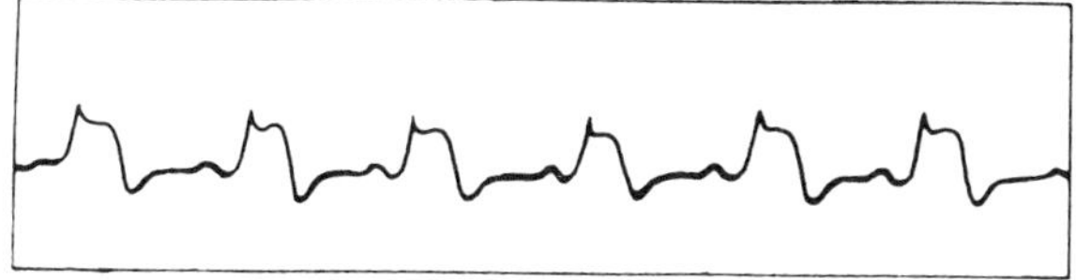

Figure 2.   Sinus rhythm at normal heart rate. Raised S–T segment.

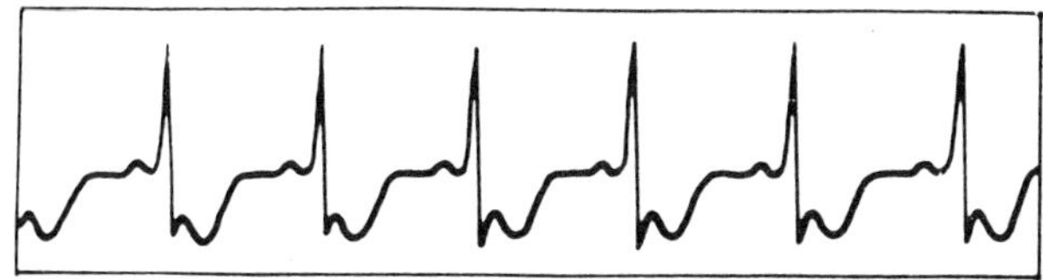

Figure. 3.   Sinus rhythm at normal heart rate. Depressed S–T segment.

Damage to the atrio-ventricular bundle results in impulses originating in the S-A node and not reaching the ventricles. This is termed 'heartblock'. However, the ventricles are made of cardiac muscle which has its own inherent rhythmicity and will continue to contract, but at a slower rate than normal. There are various degrees of this condition (Figure 4).

If another cell in the atrium originates the heartbeat this is termed 'atrial extrasystole' and this is shown as an abnormal P wave, which will be different in shape and may be inverted (Figure 5). Extrasystole may also arise from the ventricular muscle. The ECG will show an abnormally large and unusually shaped QRS complex, with no preceding P wave (Figure 6).

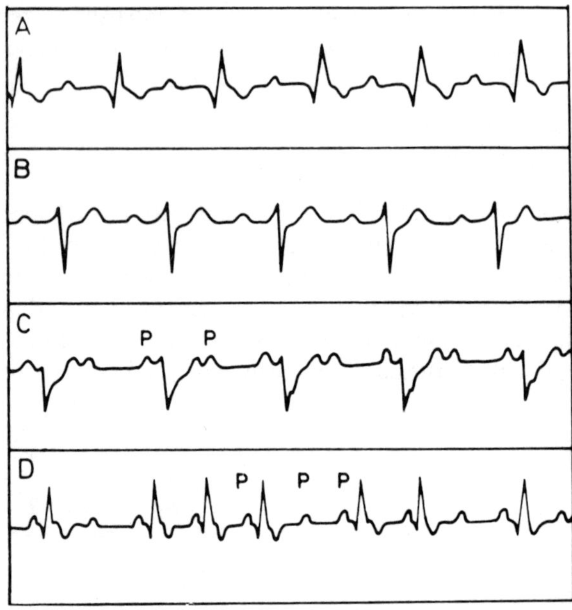

Figure 4. A and B. First degree heart block. Note length of P–R segment is constant. C. Second degree heart block. D. Second degree heart block with varying block.

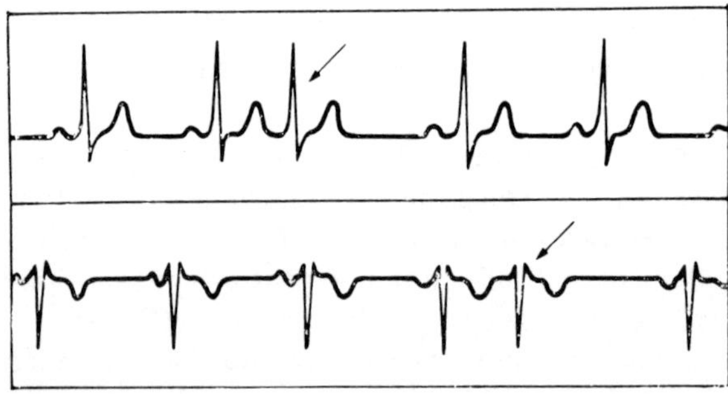

Figure 5. Atrial extrasystole. The arrows indicate an extrasystole (an extra, earlier QRS–T complex, without a preceding P wave).

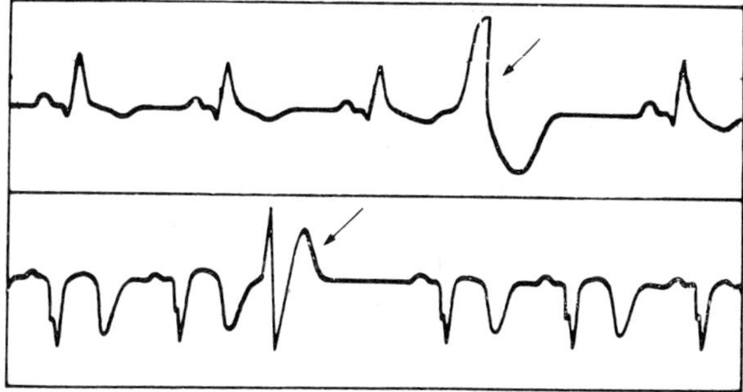

Figure 6.   Ventricular extrasystole. The arrows indicate an extrasystole (an extra, earlier QRS–T wave complex, without a preceding P wave).

There are many ectopic foci, and, therefore, no organized contraction of the ventricles as a whole. The ECG shows no organized pattern and many large abormal complexes. The danger of ventricular extrasystole is that if one falls on the upstroke of the T wave ventricular fibrillation may ensue. This results in uncoordinated ventricular activity and thus no significant cardiac output (Figure 7).

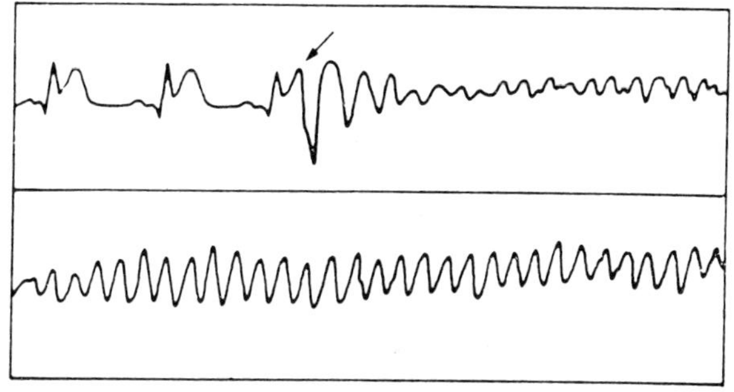

Figure 7.   Ventricular fibrillation. Ventricular extrasystole (arrow) falling on T wave ('R on T') precipitating ventricular fibrillation.

Where is the ECG performed and what preparation is necessary?

The patient must be aware that the ECG machine does not send out electric currents, but picks up the electrical changes of his heart. The patient must be asked to lay flat while the investigation is carried out and to relax with his arms by his sides and remain as still as possible. If very hirsute a local shave of the electrode sites may be required in order to achieve a clear trace.

How is the ECG performed?

Limb electrodes are applied to the right arm (R), the left arm (L) and the left leg (F). The right leg is not normally employed, but an electrode may also be applied here to earth the subject. The electrodes usually take the form of a metal plate which is strapped to the wrist and ankle with electrode jelly underneath to ensure a good electrical connection with the skin. Electrically the arms are an extension of the trunk and the electrocardiogram is a record of the voltage difference between two points. Chest electrodes are then applied which usually take the form of a suction cup which adheres to the chest. The chest leads are numbered V_1 to V_6 (Figure 8):

V_1 fourth interspace at right sternal border,

V_2 fourth interspace at left sternal border,

V_3 equidistant between V_2 and V_4,

V_4 fifth interspace in left midclavicular line,

V_5 anterior axillary line in same horizontal plane as V_4,

V_6 midaxillary line in same horizontal plane as V_4.

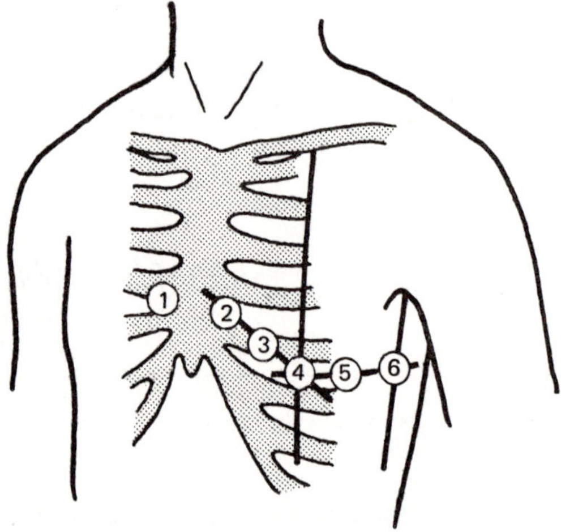

Figure 8.   Chest lead positions. 1 — at the right margin of the sternum in the 4th intercostal space; 2 — at the margin of the sternum in the 4th intercostal space; 3 — midway between positions 2 and 4; 4 — at the left midclavicular line in the 5th intercostal space; 5 — at the left anterior axillary line and at the same level as position 4; 6 — at the left midaxillary line and at the same level as position 4. (From Green (1977) Introduction to Human Physiology, 3rd edition, OUP).

What happens after the ECG?

It will only take a few minutes to complete the ECG. The areas where the electrodes have been attached should be cleaned and then the patient can resume his previous activities.

When are the results available and what might they be?

It may be possible to tell the patient straight away, but more detailed examination of the ECG tracing may delay this information for 24 hours.

Contraindications for an ECG

There are no contraindications.

Can complications occur?

There are no complications.

2.2.   Cardiac Catheterization, Echocardiography, Nuclear Imaging

What is cardiac catheterization?

Cardiac catheterization is the procedure by which a doctor passes a fine, flexible radio-opaque catheter under X-ray control into one or more of the chambers of the heart.

Why is cardiac catheterization performed?

This procedure is performed to:

1 Visualize the heart chambers and coronary arteries by means of radio-opaque substances injected into the heart under X-ray control (cardiac angiography).
2 Measure pressures and record the wave forms from the cavity of the heart chambers and the great vessels.
3 Obtain blood samples from the heart for the measurement of cardiac output and the identification of intracardiac shunting, e.g., ventricular septal defect (VSD).
4 Indicate abnormal communication by passage of a catheter.

Are there any other ways of investigating the heart function and health?

Echocardiography is a procedure using ultrasonic beams which reflect waves when they encounter boundaries between structures of different acoustic densities. The waves can be detected and used to give an electrical signal. It can be used to detect valve disorders such as calcification, vegetation or malformation, e.g., bicuspid and not tricuspid valves, pericardial effusions and the general size of the heart's cavities and muscle density.

Nuclear imaging is a quickly expanding field from which detection of infarcted tissue of the heart is possible. The isotope thallium is taken up by well perfused myocardium so that the image can show any degree of ischaemia.

Where is cardiac catheterization performed and what preparation is necessary?

The patient is usually admitted to hospital the day before cardiac catheterization so that the doctor can take a history and perform a full medical examination. In some regional centres this may be carried out on an outpatient basis. The nurse should admit the patient to the ward and record baseline observations of pulse, temperature, respiration, blood pressure, urine analysis and weight. Electrocardiogram (ECG), chest X-ray and the following blood tests are arranged: full blood count, urea and electrolytes, hepatitis screening, group and cross-matching two units of blood.

The procedure is explained to the patient and questions are encouraged and answered. The house-physician will examine the patient and a consent form will be signed. The patient should be told that the doctor may ask for deep breathing, coughing or leg raising exercises during the procedure. The night before the procedure the patient should shave the right femoral and brachial area, following which a small amount of iodine should be applied to the skin to test for allergy to the dye to be used during the procedure. Night sedation may be required. The patient should be starved for 4–6 hours previous to the procedure to ensure an empty stomach and reduce the risk of vomiting. On the day of the test glasses, false teeth and jewellery are removed and stored safely. The patient should have a bath and change into a hospital gown. A clean bed should be prepared. A premedication is given approximately 1 hour precatheterization (this may be by oral or intramuscular administration). A prophylactic antibiotic cover may also be given with the premedication.

Notes, X-rays and charts should go to the X-ray department with the patient and a nurse should stay with the patient if possible. The patient should try to micturate immediately before the investigation.

How is cardiac catheterization performed?

The patient is helped onto the X-ray table and is gently secured by straps as the table is tilted slightly from side to side. ECG leads are attached for constant monitoring (see Section 2.1). The doctor and nurse should then drape the patient with sterile towels as this is a strictly aseptic procedure. The femoral or brachial area is exposed and cleaned with iodine. If the patient is nonallergic a local anaesthetic is injected following which a small incision is made. The cardiac catheter is introduced into the vein for right-sided catheterization and the artery for left-sided catheterization. The catheter is eased along the vessels by X-ray guidance. Blood samples and pressures are taken and recorded as required.

Angiocardiography is the injection of radio-opaque dye into the chambers and great vessels of the heart and the coronary arteries. Small test doses of dye are injected when the catheter is thought to be at the origin of the coronary arteries. Once this is located a full dose is injected to show the coronary arteries. At this stage cine films are taken for studying. The patient may feel a hot flush with the administration of the dye.

When the samples and films required have been taken the doctor withdraws the catheter. With a brachial approach the incision is closed by sutures. With a femoral approach pressure is applied for about 20 min and while the patient is transferring from trolley to bed.

What happens after the cardiac catheterization?

The patient should remain on bedrest for 12 hours after brachial approach and 24 hours after femoral approach, starting off lying with one pillow and gradually sitting up a little. The affected arm or leg should be kept straight.

A normal diet may be resumed an hour after return to the ward or when the patient is fully awake. Observations are recorded as follows:

$\frac{1}{2}$-hourly pulse and blood pressure for 2 hours,

1-hourly pulse and blood pressure for 2 hours,

2-hourly pulse and blood pressure for 2 hours,

4-hourly pulse, temperature and blood pressure thereafter.

The wound should be observed at these times for oozing or signs of infection. The affected limb should also be observed for colour, warmth, sensation and peripheral pulses. If the patient experiences any tingling, numbness or pain, trained staff should be informed immediately.

The patient may appreciate a wash and change into his own night clothes. When the period of bedrest is over the patient may mobilize gently. The dressing from the brachial site should be removed on the first day postinvestigation and the sutures removed on the seventh day.

When are the results available and what might they be?

Possible findings could include the following:

1 Congenital abnormalities:

    a. Communication between left and right circulations, e.g., atrial septal defect, vetricular septal defect and persistent ductus arteriosis.
    b. Obstructive lesions, e.g., coarctation of the aorta, aortic stenosis and pulmonary stenosis.
    c. Displacement of chambers, vessels or valves.

2 Poor ventricular function and decreased cardiac output.

3 Coronary artery disease.

The doctors study the cine films and other records of tests and usually the patient is told the results within 48 hours.

Contraindications for cardiac catheterization

Recent myocardial infarction, chest pain and uncontrolled atrial fibrillation.

Can complications occcur?

Possible complications include the following:

1   Venous and arterial spasm.
2   Looping and knotting of the catheter.
3   Syncope.
4   Haemorrhage from the puncture site.
5   Dissection or perforation of the heart or of a great vessel.
6   Cardiac arrhythmias — ventricular ectopic beats, atrial ectopic beats, asystole, ventricular fibrillation.

7   Varying degrees of heartblock.

8   Tachyarrhythmias.

9   Infection.

10   Thrombophlebitis (rare).

Many of these can be effectively reduced to a minimum if the procedure is carried out with due care. Most emergencies respond to the withdrawal of the catheter to a vessel outside the heart, administration of oxygen and external cardiac massage if required. Resuscitation equipment is always available and includes oxygen, suction, d.c. fibrillator, pacemaker, thoracotomy and tracheostomy sets and emergency intravenous drugs.

Patients' comments

'I didn't find it too bad at all. I was kept busy by the doctors doing deep breathing and that kept my mind off what was going on. I was a bit worried — fear of the unknown. I thought it would only last about ¾ hour, but it took 3 hours. I only felt a bit of pain in the last ¾ hour — if felt like someone was punching me where the catheter was going in.'

'The unpleasant things I remember are a feeling of tugging and pushing in my groin and an acute pain in my head, like it was going to blow up when they pushed the dye through. However, I felt a pleasant, warm flush throughout the rest of my body. I enjoyed being able to see the catheter on the X-ray and listening to the conversation between the staff. I was a bit worried about the preparation — it looked like we were off for a major operation, but then a nurse explained why it was important to be clean and shaved and that put my mind at rest.'

'I don't remember much at all, it was a peculiar feeling and I remember having hot flushes. I just lay back and let the doctors and nurses get on with it. I remember the nice soft music playing in the background.'

'Usually I am very nervous and highly strung, but gradually what you had told me about came true. I stopped worrying when that happened. It took a long time — about 3 hours — but the doctors were nice and their chatting amused me! Also, I had a nurse I knew from the ward with me all the time.

When the dye was put in I felt like my head would explode, but it didn't last long. I felt like I was going to fall out of the bed when they tipped it to the side, but then I remembered I was strapped in. The music in the background was nice.'

2.3.   Lymphangiogram

What is a lymphangiogram?

Lymph vessels are not normally apparent on plain X-ray. Therefore a suitable radiological contrast medium must be introduced into the lymphatic system to demonstrate them. This procedure is called lymphangiography.

Why is a lymphangiogram performed?

It can be used to:

1   Determine the extent of a malignant process in the body, e.g., as part of a staging programme for Hodgkin's disease.

2   To identify lymphatically-spread metastases, e.g., in the axillary lymph nodes of a patient with carcinoma of the breast.

3   As active treatment by introducing a radioisotope into the lymphatic system, e.g., use of colloidal gold.

4   For use in benign conditions, e.g., traumatic lesions of the thoracic duct, congenital lymphoedema, tropical chyluria.

Where is the lymphangiogram performed and what preparation is necessary?

Lymphangiography is usually performed under local anaesthetic, although occasionally under general anaesthetic. It is not performed on children as their vessels are too small. It may require admission to hospital as part of a series of tests or can be done as an outpatient.

The patient always has a chest X-ray prior to the investigation. This is because the contrast medium used can cause pulmonary fibrosis, and the doctor must be aware of the condition of the patient's lungs beforehand as a baseline. The doctor may order lung function tests (see Section 7.4) if the X-ray is not satisfactory.

The patient is given a full explanation and questions are encouraged and answered. A bath or wash should be given prior to this procedure. A sedative may be given ½ hour before the lymphangiogram if it is to be under local anaesthetic. Usually diazepam 5–10 mg orally is prescribed with a good relaxing effect. The patient should empty his bladder immediately beforehand so that he can settle comfortably. If the patient is comfortable he will also be relaxed, so positioning is very important. Privacy and dignity should be maintained. He should be well supported with pillows utilizing an upturned chair in front of the backrest to bring the feet level with the end of the bed. A bedcradle draped with sterile towels is placed over the lower legs to obscure the patient's view — unless he wants to see!

Advise the patient not to wear blue nightclothes as the dye used causes skin discoloration giving a blue/grey tinge. The actual injection sites in the feet remain blue too for a week to a month, whereas general discoloration disappears in about 48 hours. Urine also turns green/blue, so this must be explained to the patient.

Some hospitals starve the patient for 4 hours prior to the investigation, to prevent nausea when the dye or contrast medium is injected. Some doctors also like the limbs to be shaved to enable thorough cleansing of the area prior to incision and thereby preventing infection.

This is not a painful investigation, but it can cause discomfort. Anxiety can be caused by the machinery used and the absolute stillness required of the patient.

How is the lymphangiogram performed?

A diffusible dye is injected into the subcutaneous tissues, usually between the toes, occasionally between the fingers. This is taken up by the lymphatics and renders them visible. The usual dye used is patent blue violet — hence the blue skin discoloration. The dispersal of the dye is assisted by walking around or by massage and limb movement for the bed-bound patient. Time taken: 10 min.

Once the vessels are demonstrated the doctor 'cuts down' and isolates the vessels (often one in each foot) he wishes to cannulate. This is a very delicate procedure as the vessels are very delicate and friable. Stay sutures are placed beneath the vessel and a minute cannula is inserted. Time taken: 30 min.

Once cannulated the radiological contrast medium is introduced, commonly oil-based, but can be water-based. When this has entered the system it remains for many months which is useful for repeat lymphangiograms which are difficult to perform because of vessel damage.

Because of the small calibre of the cannula the injection must be given slowly and at high pressure because of its viscosity. Equipment varies, but large syringes with weighted plungers are often used. Electrically driven infusion pumps may also be used. Time taken: 60–90 min.

A series of X-rays are taken using portable machines. Time taken: 5–10 min.

The nurse must ensure that an aseptic technique is employed during this procedure as any infection could be spread throughout the lymphatic system. Because of the length of the procedure (up to 3 hours) the patient will need supplies of magazines, office work and cheerful company to stave off boredom. The nurse can also assist the patient carefully on and off bedpans, offer urinals and gently treat pressure areas if necessary.

What happens after the lymphangiogram?

Once the cannula is removed, each incision is sutured or 'steristrips' are applied, with a gauze dressing. The limb is best kept elevated for 24 hours and may be painful to walk on for a few days. Analgesia should be given. Follow-up X-rays are taken the next day, including an intravenous pyelogram as the contrast medium is excreted by the kidneys, thus demonstrating any abnormality in the urinary tract if renal disease is suspected.

The incision site should be kept clean and dry, and is often slow to heal because of poor peripheral blood circulation. Sutures/steristrips are removed after 7–10 days depending on the individual.

When are the results available and what might they be?

The radiologist will report on the X-rays taken and the result is sent to the doctor. The results should be available in a few days. Possible findings include:

1   Malignant disease, particularly Hodgkin's disease and non-Hodgkin's lymphoma.

2   Lymphatically spread metastases.

3   Benign disease, e.g., traumatic lesions of the thoracic duct, congenital lymphoedema, tropical chyluria.

Contraindications for a lymphangiogram

This investigation is contraindicated in patients with lung disease.

Can complications occur?

As with the administration of any foreign substance into the lymphatics and ultimately into the bloodstream, the nurse must be aware of the danger of anaphylactic shock. This occurs if the patient has become 'sensitized' by a previous administration. The next dose causes an enormous release of histamine with resulting vasodilation and collapse. If this occurs it is an emergency situation: elevate the legs to encourage venous return, contact the doctor and maintain an airway if the patient becomes unconscious. Vasoconstricting drugs will be given immediately to revive the patient.

A lesser side-effect is a raised temperature that evening, and resulting 'flu-like' feeling showing reaction to the contrast medium. It can also cause pulmonary fibrosis as stated before.

Patients' comments

'Painful injection given between my toes. Feet painful — throbbing afterwards when local wore off. Painful to walk around for the first 2 days — feet swollen.'

2.4.   Bone Marrow Puncture

What is a bone marrow puncture?

This investigation involves the removal of red bone marrow by aspiration using a specially designed needle and guard and a trephine to remove a core of bone. A Salah needle is commonly used.

Why is a bone marrow puncture performed?

The samples are analysed in the laboratory and are used, in conjunction with a sample of peripheral blood, to diagnose blood disorders such as leukaemia, myelomas and pernicious anaemia. Treatment can be started on the basis of results gained from the samples — the procedure being repeated at intervals to assess the effectiveness of the treatment.

Where is bone marrow puncture performed and what preparation is necessary?

It can be performed on an outpatients basis, but is more commonly carried out as an inpatient. The procedure is usually carried out under local anaesthetic, although general anaesthetic may be used for young children or very anxious individuals. Multiple bone marrow aspirations are always under general anaesthetic with the resulting aspirate sent for frozen storage with a view to transplantation after aggressive therapy. If carried out under local anaesthetic a clear, careful explanation is vitally important to the patient and/or the patient's parents. This helps them prepare so that they can cooperate fully. The actual aspiration of bone marrow is painful, but if the patient is aware of this and knows that it will be relieved quickly, then he can usually cope with it. Unexpected pain has an increased intensity and will lead the bewildered patient to ask the staff 'Why didn't you tell me?'

Parents are often the best assistants for their children and can hold and comfort the child more expertly than the unfamiliar nurse. They should be encouraged to participate if they wish. Sedation is usually prescribed for children and anxious adults, e.g., diazepam.

How is bone marrow puncture performed?

The whole procedure is carried out using strict aspetic technique to minimize the risk of infection. Infection could give rise to the serious consequence of osteomyelitis, and therefore scrupulous hygiene is important.

Sites for bone marrow puncture are commonly the sternum and iliac crests in adults as they are near to the surface. The extremely obese patient may have to have the vertebrae aspirated. Young children with small bones make sternal puncture difficult as other structures may be damaged in the mediastinum, so the tibia or iliac crests may be used.

The nurse should maintain the patient's modesty and privacy and ensure he is comfortably positioned, depending on the site chosen. The patient should be encouraged to empty his bladder before the procedure. A nurse should be present to give moral support to the patient and assist the doctor. The doctor cleans the skin and then infiltrates the surrounding area with local anaesthetic so that the area becomes numb. A small incision is made and the needle introduced. The patient will feel pressure, but nothing more at this stage, as the doctor pushes through the periostium and into the bone. A syringe is attached and a sample of bone marrow aspirated. The patient will feel this as an acute pain. The doctor will then withdraw the needle and insert a wider bore needle or trephine to obtain a bone biopsy. He does this by using a 'corkscrew' action. This should not be painful but again the patient will feel increased pressure on the area. The needle is withdrawn, the specimens carefully placed on slides in suitable containers and labelled, and the area is cleaned and dressed, usually with an occlusive dressing. The whole procedure should take no longer than 5–10 min.

What happens after bone marrow puncture?

The patient may require mild analgesia to relieve soreness or aching in the area. He may be advised to rest on his bed for a short while. The dressing should be observed daily, and can be removed after 2–3 days. The wound should be kept clean and dry until completely healed.

As stated before, the patient may have to undergo further bone marrow punctures to assess treatment effectiveness. It is, therefore, very important that his first experience is a good one so that he will not dread this part of his treatment.

When are the results available and what might they be?

The doctor will need to look at the specimen, and the result should be available within 24–48 hours. Possible results include:

1 Leukaemia.
2 Myeloma.
3 Pernicious anaemia.

Contraindications for bone marrow puncture

There are no contraindications for bone marrow puncture.

Can complications occur?

1 Infection leading to osteomyelitis.
2 Haemorrhage.
3 Haematoma formation.

Patients' comments

'Varied from uncomfortable to very painful, especially when the doctor was aspirating. No problems afterwards at all. Benefited from premedication beforehand.'

Further Reading

Ashworth P and Rose H (1973) Cardiovascular Disorders, Baillière Tindall

Athayde M (1981) Interpreting the normal electrocardiogram, AORN Journal 33: 1267–1269

Becher C and Maisey M (1981) Nuclear medicine and nursing, Nursing Mirror 26 Aug: 16, 2 Sept: 34, 9 Sept: 22, 16 Sept: 32.

Bryan G (1979) Diagnostic Radiography, 3rd edition, Churchill Livingstone

Chesney D and Chesney M (1978) Care of the Patient During Radiological Procedures, 5th edition, Blackwell Scientific

Donaldson A (1981) Echocardiography: sounding out the heart, Nursing Mirror 152: 40–41

Golwin R (1981) Annual review of diagnostic imaging, Hospital Update 7: 351–357

Green J (1977) Introduction to Human Physiology, OUP

Green J (1978) Basic Clinical Physiology, 3rd edition, OUP

Greenwood D (1976) Angiography and other radiographic investigations, Nursing Times 72: 1136–1138

Guyton A (1979) Physiology in the Human Body, 5th edition, Saunders

Hamer J (1978) Introduction to electrocardiography, 2nd edition, Pitman Medical

Hoffbrand H and Pettit J (1980) Essential Haematology, Blackwell Scientific

Horrobin D (1973) Essential Physiology, MTP

Hubner P (1980) Nurse's Guide to Cardiac Monitoring, 3rd edition, Baillière Tindall

Julian D (1978) Cardiology, 3rd Edition, Baillière Tindall

Markus S (1981) Taking the fear out of bone marrow examination, Nursing (US) 11: 64–67

Stubbs D (1982) The electrocardiogram, Nursing (UK) 33: 1443–1446

Veral D (1978) Cardiac Catheterization and Angiography, 3rd edition, Churchill Livingstone

CHAPTER 3

INVESTIGATIONS ASSOCIATED WITH THE ENDOCRINE SYSTEM

The endocrine system is a complex system of ductless glands which secrete hormones (chemical messengers) directly into the circulatory system. The hormones act on various target organs and tissues and by a complex feedback mechanism a delicate balance of activity is achieved.

The system which sometimes acts with, or is influenced by, the nervous system, is one of the co-ordinating and controlling systems of the body.

The technology of endocrine hormone assay has advanced rapidly and the detail of each is beyond the scope of this book. Only a few of the investigations are included.

3.1. Oral Glucose Tolerance Test

What is an oral glucose tolerance test?

The oral glucose tolerance test measures a person's ability to stabilize his blood sugar level after taking a quantity of glucose. It consists of giving the patient a measured amount of oral glucose and the taking of blood and urine samples at regular intervals. There are recommended levels with which the results of the blood and urine samples can be compared and a diagnosis made.

Why is an oral glucose tolerance test performed?

1 In the diagnosis of diabetes mellitus.

2 To show renal glycosuria — a condition where glucose regularly and consistantly appears in the urine when the blood glucose level is less than 10 mmol/l

3 To diagnose alimentary glycosuria. This condition occurs when an unusually rapid by-transitory rise of blood glucose follows a meal and its concentration exceeds the normal renal threshold, so causing glucose to be present in the urine.

53

NOTE: The World Health Organization Committee on Diabetes in 1965 recommended that the following levels of glucose (either fasting or 2 hours after the glucose is taken) should be accepted as normal:

	Glucose concentration (mmol/l)	
Sample	*Normal*	*Diabetic*
Venous blood	6.1	7.2
Capillary blood	6.6	7.7
Plasma	7.5	8.6

In elderly persons and in patients after myocardial infarction or with malignant diseases, blood glucose concentrations may be somewhat higher than those quoted above and without the patient necessarily having diabetes mellitus.

Where is the oral glucose tolerance test performed and what preparation is necessary?

The patient should remain lying on his bed during the test. A clear, simple explanation of the test is needed in order for the patient to understand the reason for the test and what it entails. This will ensure patient cooperation. The patient should have a normal diet for the three previous days with, if possible, an unrestricted carbohydrate intake of at least 250 g. This may vary from unit to unit. This is to ensure that the test will reflect insulin response under normal dietary conditions. The patient should be allowed clear fluids only for at least 6 hours before the test.

How is the oral glucose tolerance test performed?

7.50 a.m.   A sample of urine collected and 10 ml blood taken for fasting blood sugar.

The blood may be taken by either finger prick or venesection — the doctor having introduced a butterfly cannula. This method is less traumatic for the patient.

8.00 a.m.   Glucose drink given. Oral glucose (50 g) is dissolved in 200 ml of water and given orally. The amount of glucose may vary from unit to unit. In the case of children the following formula may be used to estimate the amount:

1.75 g glucose/kg body weight.

It must be ensured that *all* the glucose is properly dissolved and diluted to the correct strength since concentration affects the absorption rate.

8.30 a.m.
9.00 a.m.
9.30 a.m.
10.00 a.m.
} Blood samples taken and urine specimens collected.

What happens after the oral glucose tolerance test?

On completion of the test the patient may be offered his normal diet and a drink. He may resume his normal activity.

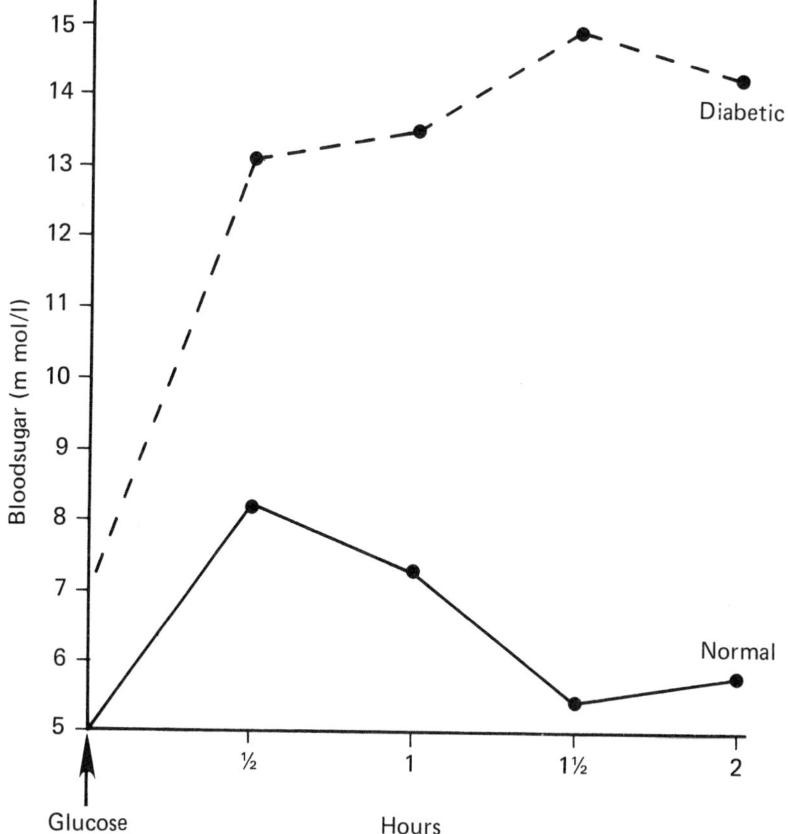

Figure 9.   Diagram to show possible results of a glucose tolerance test.

When are the results available and what might they be?

The results should be known within 24 hours. Figure 9 illustrates the results which might be obtained.

Contraindications for an oral glucose tolerance test

There are no contraindications.

Can complications occur?

There are no complications.

3.2.   Thyroid Function Tests (Radioactive Iodine Uptake and Technetium Uptake Test)

The thyroid gland consists of an isthmus and two lateral lobes, and lies in front of and on either side of the upper part of the trachea and the laminae of the thyroid cartilage.

The two main hormones produced — thyroxine (T_4) and tri-iodothyronine (T_3) — act directly on most tissues of the body to increase cellular metabolism. For these hormones to be produced, the thyroid gland utilizes iodine from the diet. Hyper- and hyposecretion of this gland has wide ranging effects on the body.

What are thyroid function tests?

Investigations of the glandular function are mainly blood tests and therefore do not cause too much distress to the patient, however anxiety can be caused when radioactivity is mentioned, for example, the radioactive iodine uptake test which makes use of the glands affinity for iodine.

Why are thyroid function tests performed?

Thyroid function tests are carried out to confirm:

1   Hyperthyroidism (thyrotoxicosis).

2   Hypothyroidism (myxoedema).

3   A 'hot' nodule, indicating malignancy.

4   The amount and distribution of active thyroid tissue.

Where are thyroid function tests performed and what preparation is necessary?

1 If clinically possible thyroid drugs are discontinued 3 days before the test.

2 The diet does not have to be altered because the amount of iodine is insignificant and therefore will not affect the results.

3 The patient will be given a hospital gown to put on as this allows ease of access to the neck.

4 The patient can be reassured that the test is painless and harmless.

5 The doctor will give the intravenous injection and the time will be recorded.

In total the test will take up to 4–5 hours but between the administration of the isotope and the scan gentle normal activities can continue.

How are radioactive iodine uptake or technetium uptake tests performed?

The patient is given an oral tracer dose of ^{131}I (half life of 8 days) or ^{132}I (half life of 2-3 hours) which will be taken up by the thyroid gland in a given time. This might be 4 hours.

This is now being superceded by the patient being given an intravenous injection of an isotope of technetium (^{99m}T) (half life of 6 hours). This gives an even smaller does of radiation which is insignificant.

At the appropriate time the patient will go to the nuclear medicine department, and the thyroid gland will be scanned to measure the amount of uptake of the isotope. A retrolinear scanner is used, which takes lifesize pictures, or a geiger counter or a sodium iodide detector may be used. The latter two do not take pictures.

What happens after the thyroid function test?

If an injection of technitium has been given, on return to the ward the patient may eat and drink normally. If ^{131}I or ^{132}I was given the patient is very slightly radioactive. However, no precautions need to be taken with regard to the radioactivity, unless for some reason the thyroid gland has not concentrated and taken up the isotope. Local policy should be consulted about this. The patient may eat and drink normally.

When are the results available and what might they be?

The results will be compiled by the physicist who will notify the patient's doctor. This may take 2–3 days. Possible findings include:

1 Hyperthyroidism (thyroitoxicosis).

2 Hypothyroidism (myxoedema).

3   A 'hot' nodule.

Other thyroid function tests involve the assay of blood specimens and are beyond the scope of this text.

Contraindications for thyroid function tests
The only contraindication to this test being performed is pregnancy.

Can complications occur?
There are no complications.

3.3.   Pancreatic Function Test

The pancreas is both an exocrine gland (producing pancreatic juices containing digestive enzymes — amylase, lipase and trypsinogen) and an endocrine gland, producing insulin and glycogen, which are necessary for the maintenance of an adequate blood sugar level.

What are pancreatic function tests?
There are two main types of pancreatic function tests:

1   Direct.
2   Indirect.

Why are pancreatic functions tests performed?

1   To measure pancreatic secretions.
2   To investigate patients with pancreatitis and possible malignancy.

1.   Direct method   This method involves the collection of pancreatic juice, which is done by performing an ERCP (see Section 1.7). It is essential that all the gastric juice is aspirated thoroughly throughout, so that uncontaminated pancreatic juice can be collected. An intravenous injection of secretin and pancreozymin is given to stimulate the pancreas, and the resultant juice is collected for assay of:

1   Volume of secretion.
2   Bicarbonate concentration.
3   Concentration of amylase and trypsinogen.

2.   Indirect method   In severe cases of pancreatic insufficiency, this may include the collection of stool specimens for steatorrhoea and creatorrhoea which may be confirmed by chemical analysis.

Also blood estimation of serum amylase levels. High levels indicate acute pancreatitis. A 24-hour urine collection to estimate amylase secretion may also be performed.

There is no special preparation for these tests.

Where is the pancreatic function test performed and what preparation is necessary?

This is the same as for an ERCP (see Section 1.7). The procedure should be explained to the patient the day before the test, and the patient should be given a chance to ask questions. The house-surgeon should then visit the patient, explain the procedure again and obtain a signed consent form. The doctor will also take blood for coagulation studies, grouping and cross-matching. The patient should be fasted for at least 8 hours prior to the test so that there is a clear picture of the stomach and duodenum in order for the ampulla of Vater to be cannulated. Immediately before the procedure the patient needs to be ready in an operation gown. Pyjama trousers should not be worn as the diathermy pad is attached to the patient's thigh. False teeth, jewellery and glasses should be removed and stored in a safe place. Notes and X-rays and the prescription chart should go to the department with the patient.

How is the pancreatic function test performed?

A silicone drink is given to the patient 5–10 min before the examination to prevent the endoscopic view being obscured by foaming. The patient should then be helped to lie comfortably in the left lateral position. They are usually turned prone when the endoscope has entered the second part of the duodenum, so this initial positioning makes it easier to move them once they are sedated. If diathermy is likely to be used, the plate is strapped to the patient's thigh at this stage.

The choice of analgesia, sedatives and local anaesthesia for the throat varies according to the doctor's preference and the patient's needs. A combination of intramuscular pethidine and diazepam and benzocaine/zylocaine spray are most commonly used. The mouth guard is then put into position and the lubricated endoscope is passed over the tongue and the patient is asked to swallow so that the endoscope passes down the oesophagus. The patient should not experience pain and discomfort is minimal if the patient is sedated.

Buscopan is given to suppress the duodenal motor activity so that the fine catheter can pass into the ampulla of Vater. The contrast medium is then slowly injected under X-ray screening. Samples are removed via the endoscope.

What happens after the pancreatic function test?

The patient will be drowsy after the procedure and should remain in bed until he is fully awake. A wash should be offered and his own night clothes be put on. Instructions sent back in the note indicate when the patient can eat and drink again, but it is usually when he is fully awake. However, if the throat has been anaesthetized then the patient should be fasted until the effects have worn off. The patient may complain of a slight sore throat, this is normal but any severe pain or feeling of distension should be reported to the doctor. Instructions about specific observations will also be given.

When are the results available and what might they be?

The doctor is usually able to tell the patient within 24–48 hours.

1   Insufficiency, that is low levels of secretion and a reduced concentration of enzymes and bicarbonate.
2   Carcinoma of the pancreas.
3   Stone in the bile duct.

Contraindications for the pancreatic function test

There are a few contraindications for this test; they include severe heart disease, recent myocardial infarction, severe respiratory disease, including active tuberculosis, and a positive blood test for Australian antigen.

Can complications occur?

Complications are rare but the following may occur:

1.   Sore throat.
2.   Venous thrombosis.
3.   Respiratory suppression due to oversedation or inhalation of secretions.
4.   Shock due to perforation or bleeding.
5.   Blurred vision or retention of urine due to large doses of buscopan.

3.4.   Adrenal Function — Vanillylmandelic Acid (VMA) Test

What is a VMA test?

A 24-hour collection of urine for vanillylmandelic acid (VMA) may be performed if an adrenal medullary tumour (phaeochromocytoma) is suspected (see Section 8.5). As this tumour secretes excessive amounts of adrenaline and noradrenaline into the bloodstream, this leads to an excess of catecholamines in the urine, including VMA. Normally less than 150 μg are excreted per day.

What preparation is necessary?

In order for an accurate result to be obtained, the patient needs to be given a vanilla-free diet (i.e., no tea, coffee, bananas, sweets or tomatoes) for at least 48 hours before the test.

   Methyldopa (Aldomet) should not be given for at least a week before the test, and any other drugs being taken should be noted on the request form.

How is the test performed?

The urine is collected in a container containing 20 ml of hydrochloric acid as a preservative.

When are the results available?

Results are available in 2–3 days.

Further Reading

Bonar J (1980) Diabetes, 2nd edition, Kimpton

Ireland J (1980) Diabetes Today, HM&M

MacLeod J (editor) (1981) Davidson's Principles and Practice of Medicine, 13th edition, Churchill Livingstone

McCulloch J (1981) Biochemistry: blood glucose tests, Nursing Mirror 152: 36–37

McCulloch J (1982) Biochemistry: assessment of thyroid function, Nursing Mirror 154: 34

Nursing Times (1979) Systems of Life 57: Adrenal Glands 2, Nursing Times Supplement

Sykes M (1981) Aspects of Gastroenterology for Nurses, Pitman Medical

WHO (1980) Diabetes Mellitus, Technical Report Series No 646, WHO

CHAPTER 4

INVESTIGATIONS USED IN GYNAECOLOGY

The female genital organs include the ovary and uterine (fallopian) tube on each side and in the midline the uterus and vagina.

Any disease and trauma to this system can cause physical problems of pain, discomfort, haemorrhage or unpleasant discharges. Psychological problems arise not only for the patient who may feel that her fertility and femininity may be at risk but also for her partner and the family.

Included in this section are investigations which may be carried out on the breasts. The breasts (mammary glands) are found on the anterior wall of the thorax, and consist of glandular and fatty tissue. Changes in the size and type of tissue occur first at puberty and then under the influence of the hormones of the menstrual cycle. The development of the breasts and other secondary sexual characteristics is the outward sign that puberty has been reached. Again any disease or trauma to the breasts will cause both physical and psychological problems.

Therefore any investigations must be sensitively approached and carried out. Privacy, dignity and confidentiality must be maintained at all times.

4.1. Cervical Smears

Gynaecology is the area of medicine concerned with the female reproductive system. It is an emotionally delicate area in which even the most routine examination or investigation can be a daunting prospect for a patient. The role of the nurse is important in giving the patient emotional support and comfort, and chaperoning the male doctor.

Whenever a male doctor examines a patient internally in the course of a gynaecological examination, he must have a female present to act as a chaperone. This duty is part of the nurse's overall care of her patient. She has a dual function as a chaperone; first, to the patient to give her psychological support, and second to the doctor to give him professional support.

What is a cervical smear?

A cervical smear should be carried out routinely on all women over the age of 20 at regular intervals. It is a means of detecting the presence of cervical carcinoma, even at an early asymptomatic stage. The cervix is exposed by insertion of a vaginal speculum and cervical epithelial cells are obtained by scraping the cervix with a spatula. The patient should not experience any pain from this procedure although she may feel pressure when the sample is being obtained. The cells obtained are then smeared onto a microscope slide, covered with microscopic fixative and sent to the laboratory for examination.

Why is a cervical smear performed?

Cervical cancer is now known to be linked with sexual activity, therefore, any sexually active female should have cervical smears taken regularly. The incidence of the disease increases with age. At some centres two annual cervical smears are taken and then if the woman has no evidence of disease, i.e., no positive smears, the cervical smear will be repeated at 2-yearly intervals. The medical profession vary in their opinion as to how often cervical smears should be taken.

Where is the cervical smear performed and what preparation is necessary?

Below are a few points to remember when assisting with an internal examination. In practice you will be shown the technical skills needed for assisting with the examination, and perhaps taking a cervical smear for cytology or a high vaginal swab for bacteriology by another member of the nursing staff. You will also have to be adaptive to the requests of individual doctors.

Before the examination give a detailed explanation of what is involved to the patient. Explain that you are going to be present. Some patients associate the examination with the sexual act. They should be assured that it is purely a clinical examination. Ask the patient to pass urine before the examination and whether she has a tampon or cap still in situ. Ask if she has ever had a previous examination. If she is menstruating the examination may be postponed.

Ensure complete privacy. Draw curtains fully and keep them closed. Keep as much as possible of the body covered with a blanket. Talk to the patient in a lowered voice to avoid the feeling that everyone else in the ward can hear.

How is the cervical smear performed?

Position the patient comfortably and remove all clothing from the waist downwards. Lie her on her back with one or two pillows only. When the examination takes place she will either put her feet up in the stirrups if on a gynaecological examination couch, or if in bed will draw her legs up, feet together and flat, and let her knees flop apart. If it is impossible for her to be positioned in this way then a lateral position may be used. This may be the case if disease of the hips or knees is present causing painful or limited movement.

The doctor will work from the right-hand side of the patient. The examination trolley should be on the same side of the bed as the doctor.

Throughout the examination face the head of the patient. It helps her realize you are more interested in her as a person than the examination. Talk to her, hold her hand or do anything that will help her to relax. Maintain her modesty at all times. Be ready to assist the doctor in passing and lubricating instruments, etc., as he directs.

The doctor will stand on the right-hand side of the patient (or at the foot of the examination couch if the patient has her feet in stirrups). He will palpate the abdominal organs and examine the external genitalia for abnormalities. The mucous secreting Bartholins glands at the opening of the vagina can easily be infected causing a Bartholins abscess. This is usually drained surgically under anaesthetic.

To examine the internal pelvic organs a warmed speculum (usually Cusco's or Sims') is passed into the vagina and then opened in order to give clear viewing of the cervix. The speculum should be lubricated with jelly prior to insertion and the patient encouraged to relax. It sometimes feels uncomfortable, but should not be painful unless the vaginal walls are inflamed due to infection. With the speculum in place the cervix can be viewed and swabs and smears taken for investigation. High vaginal swabs when cultured may show the presence of vaginal infection or sexually transmitted diseases.

What happens after the cervical smear?

At the end of the examination give the patient tissues to wipe herself dry. Help her to dress again if necessary. Depending on local procedure wash and resterilize the speculum used or return it to the central sterile supplies department for resterilization. Ensure that any specimens taken are correctly labelled, sent to the appropriate place and recorded in the Kardex.

When are the results available and what might they be?

The patient should be informed of the results if any abnormality is detected. This may be within a few days or longer, depending on how quickly the results are obtained.

Contraindications for a cervical smear

There are no contraindications.

Can complications occur?

There are no complications.

Patients' comments

'It wasn't painful at all. I felt the speculum — nothing else.'

'I didn't feel any discomfort perhaps because I was relaxed. It is important to relax and think about something else.'

4.2. Laparoscopy

What is a laparoscopy?

This is an investigatory operation performed under general anaesthetic. It involves looking into the abdominal and pelvic cavities via a laparoscope, after the abdomen has been distended with carbon dioxide, or a mixture of nitrogen and air, to make viewing easier.

Why is a laparoscopy performed?

Laparoscopy is performed to investigate the cause of amenorrhoea, dysmenorrhoea, dyspareunia, infertility, pain or swellings in the pelvis. It can also be used for sterilization as the fallopian tubes can be diathermied or clipped off via the laparoscope.

Sometimes dye is used to check the patency of the fallopian tubes. Dye is inserted via the vagina and with the patient in a head down lying position, the distal end of the fallopian tubes are observed via the laparoscope for spillage of the dye. Adhesions in the tubes prevent the dye reaching the ovaries and helps explain a cause of infertility. During the operative procedure the uterus, ovaries and other pelvic and abdominal organs can be observed for abnormalities and malfunction.

Where is a laparoscopy performed and what preparation is necessary?

Usually a patient will be asked to come into hospital the day before the laparoscopy and will be able to be discharged, if no postoperative complications occur and the patient feels well, the day following the procedure. In some centres it can be done on a day outpatient basis.

On admission a set of baseline observations of temperature, pulse, respiration and blood pressure should be recorded, the patient weighed and a urine analysis performed routinely to ensure that the patient is fit for anaesthesia.

Specific preinvestigations include:

1   Full medical and gynaecological history and examination by the doctor, including an internal pelvic examination.

2   A high vaginal swab is taken if any signs of infection are noted.

3   Blood sampling for haemoglobin levels, grouping and serum in case of a necessary further operative procedure.

4   A clear bowel should be ensured.

5   An abdominal shave is performed to remove any hair around the umbilicus and pelvic shave to remove the top 2 cm of pubic hair. Both of these are carried out to help prevent infection.

6   The patient is starved for 6 hours prior to the investigation.

7   A full explanation should be given and written consent to the investigation must be obtained from the patient. If sterilization is to be performed the husband or partner should be involved too. Questions should be encouraged and answered.

8   The patient has a bath, clean linen and operation gown to minimize infection risk just prior to the premedication being given.

9   The premedication is usually given as for any general anaesthetic.

How is the laparoscopy performed?

Laparoscopy is performed in an operating theatre after the patient has been anaesthetized. It takes about 15 min to perform. After the patient has been covered in sterile towels and the abdominal skin prepared with antiseptic lotion a small incision is made below the umbilicus for insertion of the laparoscope (a telescopic instrument with attached fibreoptic viewer and light source). A puncture hole is also made and carbon dioxide or nitrogen and air is pumped into the abdominal cavity to distend it (usually about 3 litres are used). Sometimes both the gas and the laparoscope enter via the same incision. The patient's head is lowered so that the pelvic organs fall more into the abdominal cavity. Full examination is made of the organs and the patency of the fallopian tubes tested with dye if necessary. At this stage if the laparoscopy is being performed for therapeutic reasons, e.g., clip sterilization, the procedure is carried out. The laparoscope is removed, the gas released from the abdominal cavity and the incision closed with a suture, usually black silk type, and covered with elastoplast (note should have been made if the patient is allergic to elastoplast preoperatively).

What happens after the laparoscopy?

When the patient reurns to the ward following a laparoscopy she will need the full postoperative care for minor general surgery, including maintenance of airway, observations, control and relief of pain and nausea. Specific care includes:

1   Half-hourly observation of colour, pulse, blood pressure, vaginal loss, wound loss, until her condition is stable, but for at least 2 hours. Temperature is to be checked every 4 hours unless hyperpyrexia occurs. If dye has been used the vaginal loss will be blue/green in colour and can be heavy. A sanitary towel should be kept in place to avoid getting dye on clothes as it stains. When a sanitary towel is changed ensure that vaginal loss has been recorded.

2   There are no restrictions on drinking and eating once the patient is conscious and not nauseated.

3   Vulval toilet should be performed as a socially clean procedure as it is not the site of the operation. Warm water or saline and cotton wool should be adequate.

4   Pain experienced after this investigation varies from one person to another. Patients can experience referred pain to the shoulder from remaining gas pressing on the diaphragm and irritating the phrenic nerve. Analgesia prescribed may include narcotics intramuscularly, e.g., omnopon 10 mg or pethidine 50 mg, although these are not usually required since oral analgesia seems adequate. Pain may persist for several days.

5   Observe for when the patient first passes urine. Urine retention should not occur. If dye has been used the urine will often appear blue/green and the patient needs to be forewarned about this.

6   If there are sutures in the incisions these can be removed if the wound has healed and new elastoplast applied if necessary. In some centres the suture may be removed 24 hours later or in the outpatients department up to 7 days later.

Discharge from hospital can usually take place on the first postoperative day, unless there are complications or a slow recovery from anaesthesia. An outpatients clinic appointment may be necessary, depending on the reason for laparoscopy.

Return to work takes place when the patient feels able. A sedentary worker should be able to return to work after 3 or 4 days. Someone with an active job may need longer away from work.

Sexual relationships can begin again when the patient feels comfortable enough for such.

When are the results available and what might they be?

The doctor may be able to tell the patient these within 24 hours. If specimens have been sent to the laboratory for further tests there may be a delay of a few days until the results are available. Possible findings include:

1   Ovarian cysts.
2   Tubal abnormalities.
3   Adhesions.
4   Congenital abnormalities.

Contraindications for a laparoscopy

There are no specific contraindications.

Can complications occur?

Occasionally patients may have a general postoperative or postanaesthetic complication, but as the anaesthetic is quite mild the patient usually recovers well. Specific complications include:

1   Bleeding from incisions. The wounds should be checked regularly as bleeding can be quite heavy and an extra suture may be needed.
2   Pain can be quite severe sometimes due to bruising or bleeding into the abdominal region or vagina.
3   Distension and flatus may persist for a few days due to the presence of residual gas.

Patients' comments

'When I came to on the ward I felt very sleepy and was able to doze for most of the afternoon. My tummy was sore and felt distended — pain killing tablets helped.'

'I did not feel much pain, but felt distended with a lot of wind. I had to wear a sanitary towel for 2 days afterwards because of the discharge. I went home the day after the operation.'

'It was a minor operation and things went well. I had a light supper that day and was even out of bed in the evening. I went home the next day.'

'I was sterilized. It was not painful, but I did feel sore for a few days. It was worth it though.'

4.3.   Thermography

What is thermography?

All tissues of the body produce heat from metabolic activity. In areas of rapid cell division, as in a malignant growth, this is greatly increased. By using a thermographic scanner that is heat sensitive it is able to build up a pictorial record of the infrared radiation emitted. It is a noninvasive investigation and as ionizing radiation is not involved is very safe.

Why is thermography performed?

Thermography is performed to aid diagnosis of a lump in the breast.

Where is thermography performed and what preparation is necessary?

It is carried out mainly in breast-screening clinics or special centres. There is no preparation for this test, except explaining the procedure to the patient.

How is thermography performed?

The patient is asked to strip to the waist and remove any jewellery from around her neck. She then sits in an air-conditioned cubicle at a cool temperature of 19°C. Her arms should be above her head to allow the axillary tail of the breast to cool. This may be for 15 min or so.

The patient will then be asked to sit in an upright chair with her arms resting on side arm-rests. Three scans will be taken:

1   Anterior view.

2   Two lateral views for accuracy of diagnosis.

The whole test should not take more than 20 min from commencement to completion.

What happens after thermography?

The patient dresses again, and can go home.

When are the results available and what might they be?

Diagnosis can be difficult due to hormone activity, lactation, recent surgery, trauma or skin conditions. The results should be available within a few days, and may indicate the presence of a lump in the breast.

Contraindications for thermography

There are no contraindications for thermography.

Can complications occur?

There are no complications associated with thermography.

Patients' comments

'Embarrassing to sit half naked in a cold room beforehand, but otherwise no complaints.'

4.4.   Mammography

What is a mammogram?

A mammogram is an X-ray taken of the breast. It is carried out on women when clinical examination or thermography reveals a suspicious lump in the breast.

Why is a mammogram performed?

Special X-ray equipment is used to visualize both the skin of the breast and the chest wall, so that an accurate diagnosis can be made. When used by experts diagnosis of breast lumps can be up to 75% accurate using a mammogram.

Where is a mammogram performed and what preparation is necessary?

This test may be carried out in X-ray departments and in well women's screening clinics. No preparation is necessary, except the explanation of the procedure to the patient.

How is a mammogram performed?

The patient is asked to stand up, resting the breast on an X-ray plate and then a number of pictures from different views are taken. Some compression of the breast is necessary, which can be uncomfortable for the patient. The X-ray pictures taken may show opacities, calcification and enlarged lymph nodes, which may alert the doctor to a malignancy which may have been overlooked on clinical examination. The whole procedure should last less than 20 min.

When are the results available and what might they be?

The results should be available within a few days, and will confirm the presence or absence of a lump in the breast.

Contraindications for a mammogram

There are no contraindications for a mammogram.

Can complications occur?

There are no complications associated with mammography.

Patients' comments

'Uncomfortable when breast is squashed and compressed, but otherwise no side-effects or problems.'

Further Reading

Barnes J (1980) Lecture Notes in Gynaecology, 4th edition, Blackwell Scientific

Garrey M (1978) Gynaecology Illustrated, 2nd edition, Churchill Livingstone

Phillip E (1982) Pass the laparoscope, World Medicine, 20 March 1982, 88–92

Shorthouse M and Brush M (1981) Gynaecology in Nursing Practice, Baillière Tindall

Weir J and Abrahams P (1978) Atlas of Radiological Anatomy, Pitman Medical

White L (1979) Cancer Screening and Detection Manual for Nurses, McGraw Hill

Wilcox P (1981) Benign breast disorders, American Journal of Nursing 81: 1644–1645

CHAPTER 5

INVESTIGATIONS ASSOCIATED WITH THE MUSCULOSKELETAL SYSTEM

The musculoskeletal system forms the framework of the human body and by its specialized nature enables very complex and co-ordinated activity to take place. It is dependent on a healthy nervous system for its effective activity but, like all systems in the body, is reliant on normal homoeostasis.

Conditions affecting the system are often painful and disabling, so accurate early diagnosis is important if disruption of normal activities is to be minimized.

5.1. Arthroscopy

What is an arthroscopy?

Arthroscopy is an endoscopic investigation usually performed under a general anaesthetic to examine the internal structures of a joint. It is a recent technique, which at present is confined to examination of the knee.

Why is an arthroscopy performed?

Arthroscopy can be performed for diagnosing and assessing the reasons for joint pain which may be due to:

1 Rheumatoid arthritis.

2 Osteoarthrosis.

3 The presence of loose or foreign bodies.

4 Chondromalacia patellae.

5 Chronic synovitis.

6 Tuberculosis.

7 Internal derangement of the knee.

It can also be used for therapeutic purposes, removal of small loose or foreign bodies, biopsy of synovial membrane and removal of part of the meniscus.

Where is the arthroscopy performed and what preparation is necessary?

Usually a patient will be asked to come into hospital the day before the arthroscopy, and be able to be discharged, if no further operative procedure is performed and if there are no complications, the day after the investigation. In some centres this investigation may be carried out on a day-case basis.

On admission a set of baseline observations of temperature, pulse, respiration and blood pressure should be recorded, and the patient weighed and a urine analysis performed routinely in preparation for an anaesthetic.

Specific preinvestigation preparations include:

1   Full medical history and examination of the knees by a doctor.
2   Plan X-rays of affected knee, tunnel view and skyline view of patella.
3   Possibly a previous arthrogram.
4   Blood sampling for a full blood count.
5   Patient must give written consent to the investigation and the affected limb must be marked by a doctor.
6   Ensure that there are no cuts or abrasions of the skin around the knee. Shave any hair from the area of incision (according to the surgeon's preference) in order to minimize the risk of infection.
7   Preinvestigation physiotherapy to encourage quadriceps exercises.
8   Antiseptic bath or skin preparation prior to operation. Patient then wears an operation gown.
9   Premedication is given as for any general anaesthetic.

How is the arthroscopy performed?

Once the patient is anaesthetized a tourniquet is applied at the thigh to reduce blood flow to the joint. The skin is prepared with antiseptic lotion and the leg draped in such a way that the assistant can manipulate the leg and remain sterile.

A small incision is made in the infrapatellar region and the cannula of the arthroscope is pushed through the incision into the joint space. A fibreoptic light source and an irrigation of physiological saline is attached to the arthroscope. The knee is extended with the saline, usually 100–200 ml and the internal structures of the joint viewed. A second trocar and cannula may be introduced for use of biopsy forceps, if a biopsy is to be performed or a foreign body is to be removed.

At the end of the procedure, if no further steps are to be taken, the saline is drained, the arthroscope removed and the incision closed with one suture, usually prolene. A sterile dressing and crepe bandage are applied and the tourniquet removed. Before leaving theatre the toes should be checked for circulation.

The procedure will take 30 min minimum, but much longer if operative procedures are carried out.

What happens after an arthroscopy?

Following an arthroscopy a patient will need the usual postoperative care for minor general surgery, including maintenance of airway, observation, control and relief of pain and nausea, etc. Once conscious the patient may appreciate a wash and can change into his own night clothes. Specific care includes:

1 Regular observations of pulse and blood pressure every ½ hour for at least the first 2 hours. Temperature recordings every 4 hours, unless hyperpyrexial.

2 Observation of the dressing to check for oozing of the wound.

3 Checking of toes for circulation and sensation to ensure there was no surgical trauma to blood or nerve supply and that post-traumatic oedema does not occlude these pathways.

4 Elevate the foot of the bed to help prevent postsurgical oedema.

5 Encourage the patient to 'straight leg raise' and thus exercise his quadricep muscles.

6 The patient can drink and eat when fully awake, if he does not feel nauseated.

7 Pain may be experienced after the procedure, but is usually controlled by a moderate oral analgesic.

8 Patients are encouraged to remain in bed resting and then are mobilized with a walking stick the following day, or the evening of the same day if their procedure was performed in the morning.

NOTE: Some hospitals, however, may not keep a patient in overnight. The investigation can, if necessary, be performed under local anaesthetic.

9   The suture is usually removed 7–10 days later by the patient's own general practitioner or at an outpatients clinic.

10   Discharge from hospital usually takes place the following day, unless there are any immediate complications.

When are the results available and what might they be?

The doctor will be able to tell the patient the results straight away. Possible findings include:

1   Rheumatoid arthritis.

2   Osteoarthritis.

3   The presence of loose or foreign bodies.

4   Chondromalacia patellae.

5   Chronic synovitis.

6   Tuberculosis.

7   Internal derangement of the knee.

Contraindications for an arthroscopy

There are no contraindications.

Can complications occur?

Complications are very rare — the investigation is straightforward and if the patient tolerates a general anaesthetic satisfactorily he will usually make a good recovery. Possible complications include:

1   Excessive swelling or effusion.

2   Introduction of infection.

3   Injury to cartilage or capsule.

4   Traumatic arthritis in the long-term

Patients' comments

'It was very straightforward. I was in hospital for 3 days and walked out without any problems. I understand that in America they can do this on an outpatient basis.'

'I did not really feel any pain, just a soreness. I left hospital the next day, without even a walking stick!'

'The anaesthetic had been fairly light. I did not have any problems with nausea and was able to eat a light meal 3 to 4 hours after the operation.'

'Following my arthroscopy I was told that I would need further surgery — a synovectomy — because my knee was affected with rheumatoid arthritis. I was given a date for readmission before leaving. Sometimes further surgery can be done at the same time.'

5.2.   Myelography and Radiculography

What is a myelogram?

This investigation is performed using a contrast medium which is introduced via a lumbar puncture into the spinal canal and its flow monitored on camera and then spinal X-rays are taken at relevant points in the procedure. It is usually performed under local anaesthesia.

Why is a myelogram performed?

By outlining the spinal theca it is possible to detect and establish the position of lesions which may be compressing the spinal cord and/or spinal nerves.

Where is the myelogram performed and what preparation is necessary?

A full explanation is given to the patient and a consent form signed. The diagnostic X-ray department will send a preparation instruction slip to the ward the day before the investigation is planned. Fasting is not necessary, but only a light meal should be taken if possible not less than 4 hours before the test. This avoids faintness during what may be a very long procedure of 1–2 hours.

Scrupulous cleanliness of the lumbar puncture site should be ensured to minimize the risk of infection. A local shave may be required if the area is very hirsute. After a bath or wash a clean gown should be provided. Premedication is not usually required, but a very anxious patient may be given diazepam orally. This is often the drug of choice and helps reduce anxiety and so enables the patient to cooperate.

In the case of old age, spinal injury or neurological disease, when the patient's mobility may be restricted, the process can be painful and prolonged. It is important that appropriate analgesia is given before and during the procedure.

How is the myelogram performed?

The patient will arrive at the department on a trolley or in a wheelchair. He is transferred onto the X-ray table and the lumbar puncture is either carried out with the patient lying on his left side or lying prone. The ambulant patient is sometimes positioned in a comfortable sitting position for lumbar puncture. Local anaesthesia is introduced and the lumbar puncture is performed (see Section 6.4 on lumbar puncture). A small amount of cerebrospinal fluid is removed and then the contrast medium is slowly introduced. The sample of cerebrospinal fluid is put into numbered and labelled bottles and are returned to the ward with the patient in case they are required for further tests.

The contrast mediums which may be used are:

1   Metrizamide (Amipaque), a water soluble, non-ionic compound, is most often used as it produces fewer complications and is absorbed within 24 hours.

2   Myodil (Iophendylate injection) is an iodine-based, pale yellow, oily substance reserved only to investigate obstructive cord compression, mostly in patients with spinal metastases or rheumatoid arthritis. It is not easily absorbed — 1 ml/year. Consequently, as much of the medium is withdrawn at the end of the investigation as possible.

Next a picture is taken and developed to ensure that the medium is in place before a more comprehensive series are taken with the patient now lying on the X-ray table. Since the medium is heavier than cerebrospinal fluid it is encouraged to move along the spinal canal by tilting the table. Visual fluoroscopic control is used by the radiographer to control the tilt.

Although the patient is well secured in a harness and cannot fall the patient will feel reassured if a nurse can either hold his hand or stay within his range of vision whilst the X-rays are being taken. The tilting of the table can be compared to a slow motion fair ride which can be quite alarming, especially to older patients. Giddiness and even nausea are common symptoms whilst undergoing myelography, hence the need for a time lapse since the last meal.

What happens after the myelogram?

When collecting the patient from the radiography department always check whether it has been performed under a local or general anaesthetic, the type of contrast medium used and specific instructions for postinvestigation care regarding positioning of the patient and observations.

For water soluble myelography (radiculography) — metrizamide (Amipaque)   Before leaving the department the ambulant patient is put in the sitting position for a few minutes to allow the contrast medium to move into the lumbar region.

On the ward the patient should be nursed with the head raised on two pillows for 6 hours (remind the patient not to bend down as it would result in severe headache due to the contrast medium running into the brain — so ensure that male patients have a urinal at an appropriate height). A wash may be appreciated. A further 24 hours of bedrest is advised. The dye will have been completely absorbed within a couple of days. Neurological observations should be recorded:

½-hourly for 2 hours,

1-hourly for 4 hours,

4-hourly for 12 hours, provided the observations are satisfactory.

These should also include assessment of sensation, warmth and mobility of lower limbs.

For oil-based myodil myelography   This medium is not easily absorbed so the patient is required to be nursed flat with one pillow beneath the head for 24 hours. This avoids headache. Neurological observations should be recorded for:

½-hourly for 2 hours,

2-hourly for 4 hours,

4-hourly for 12 hours, provided the observations are satisfactory.

Limb assessment should also be carried out.

In both cases food and drink can be taken as required, but nausea may be experienced so small meals may be advisable and antiemetics prescribed and given.

When are the results available and what might they be?

The results should be available within 2–3 days as soon as the radiologist has looked at the X-rays and sent a report to the doctor. Possible findings may include:

1   Lesions of vertebrae.
2   Lesions of the spinal cord or spinal nerves.

3   Congenital abnormalities.

4   Prolapsed intervertebral disc.

Contraindications for a myelogram

Contraindications could include:

1   A history of epilepsy is considered to be a relative contraindication to the use of both media.

2   Patients receiving drugs, especially of the phenothiazine group, should have these drugs withheld for 48 hours prior to myelography.

3   Special care should be taken with alcoholics and drug addicts.

Can complications occur?

There is a risk of introducing infection when performing the lumbar puncture so strict aseptic precautions must be adhered to throughout the procedure.

All procedures using contrast media can cause adverse reactions in the form of hypersensitivity when epileptic-type fits can be induced. A test dose should be given prior to the total injection. These risks should be pointed out to the patient and relatives, but at the same time reassure them by explaining that if there is any hint of an allergic reaction then the dye is immediately removed and the appropriate antidote given. Pain is not common. Headache, however, is not uncommon and appropriate analgesia should be given.

Arachnoiditis is a major complication with the oil-based contrast medium. This causes lumber or sacral nerve root pain, which may persist for weeks or months.

Patients' comments

'Once I was actually in the investigation room all my fears were taken away as everything was explained to me as the investigation was done. The staff explanations put me at rest.'

'My back was cleaned and then they froze it. I felt a prick in my back as they injected the dye. I was in a curled-up position on the table — as you would be in mother's womb — hands and legs in a ball. Slowly they tipped the table until I was standing up. I wasn't worried, although it was a strange sensation, because there was a firm foot rest on the end of the table and two knobs above me to hold on to so I knew I was safe. In this position the X-rays were taken at all different angles. I was told the result at once and so I had no awful worrying time.'

'The investigation was fine — no problems. I knew that sometimes headaches may occur afterwards, but the staff explained that I was to lie flat 24 hours afterwards. I did this and had no problems. I do know that sometimes, depending on the dye, you may need to first sit up for 6 hours and then stay in your bed 24 hours. I also was told to drink much water because fluid was taken away from the spine. So I did drink lots of orange squash.'

Further Reading

Chapman S and Nakielny R (1981) Guide to Radiological Procedures, Baillière Tindall

Crawford Adams J (1981) Outline of Orthopaedics, 9th edition, Churchill Livingstone

Cyriax J and Russell G (1978) Textbook of Orthopaedic Medicine, 7th edition, Baillière Tindall

Hall H (1981) The Back Doctor, Gollanz

Kanes G (1981) History and development of the arthroscope, Natnews 18: 45–48

Lamb S (1978) Nurse's changing role in water soluble myelography, J Neurosurg Nursing 10: 189–190

Weir J and Abrahams P (1978) Atlas of Radiological Anatomy, Pitman Medical

CHAPTER 6

INVESTIGATIONS ASSOCIATED WITH THE NERVOUS SYSTEM

The nervous system consists of the central, peripheral and autonomic systems. Together they form one of the main co-ordinating and controlling systems of the body. Nervous tissue consists of nerve cells, which once damaged cannot regenerate, and myelinated and non-myelinated nerve fibres.

Nervous tissue is delicate and easily damaged by disease, trauma or drugs. Very slight alteration in its healthy state will result in wide ranging effects on the persons ability to function 'normally'.

Investigations of neurological dysfunction are highly technical and in some cases not without risk, although modern techniques like computerized axial tomography have reduced some of the potential dangers to the patient.

It is therefore very important that nurses are aware of this and are able to prepare patients for these investigations correctly, to monitor their condition and to care for them postinvestigation.

6.1. Airencephalogram (AEG)

What is an airencephalogram (AEG)?

In an airencephalogram 25–60 ml of air are injected into the cerebrospinal fluid surrounding the spinal cord using the same procedure as a lumbar puncture (see Section 6.4), i.e., between the third and fourth or fourth and fifth lumbar vertebrae. When the patient is placed in a sitting position the air rises to the ventricles and will show up on the X-ray. Depending on the position of the patient different ventricles are filled with air and for this reason the position of the patient is changed by the movements of the table to which they are firmly strapped.

The procedure is generally carried out under general anaesthetic, as it is painful and very bewildering to be turned upside down and into the other positions that the table can adopt. It may also be performed under local anaesthesia.

82

Why is an AEG performed?

To identify cause of headache, flashing lights and parasthesia. To aid differential diagnosis of acromegaly or hypopituitarism, to visualize tumours and to assess the extent of hydrocephalus. It may be used as a diagnostic tool in a young patient to confirm dementia. This investigation is usually not performed when intracranial pressure is raised.

Where is the AEG performed and what preparation is necessary?

The patient is admitted 1–2 days prior to the investigation so that full assessment for suitability for general anaesthesia can be carried out. Baseline observations should be taken of temperature, pulse and respiration, and full neurological observations may also be required. A full explanation is given and the consent form signed. On the day of investigation the patient is prepared as for a general anaesthetic. The local preparation of the lumbar puncture site should be checked. A nurse should accompany the patient to the X-ray department where the investigation will take place.

How is the AEG performed?

The patient is anaesthetized and an endotracheal tube is inserted to maintain the airway. An intravenous infusion is commenced. A lumbar puncture is performed (see Section 6.4) and the patient then sat up by adjusting the table into a 'chair'. A space at the back of the table enables the doctor to reach the lumbar puncture site. About 6 ml of cerebrospinal fluid is withdrawn and then 5–30 ml of air or oxygen is introduced. The patient is securely strapped down to the table which is then rotated, the patient may be turned upside down, this is to ensure that the air circulates thoroughly throughout the ventricular spaces, thus visualizing any lesions and abnormalities present. Movement of the table is necessarily slow because the patient is anaesthetized and has the intravenous infusion in progress, so the whole procedure may take up to 2 hours for all necessary X-rays to be taken.

What happens after the AEG?

The patient may remain in the X-ray department until fully conscious or return to the ward (see local policy). For the first 24 hours the patient must lie flat with one pillow to reduce the risk of headache due to raised intracranial pressure caused by the air. After 24 hours the patient may be raised to a semisitting position, and after 48 hours, if the patient's condition is satisfactory, he can begin to be mobilized gradually. Close observations must be carried out for signs of altered neurological state, especially intracranial pressure indicated by raised blood pressure and falling pulse rate (some degree will be present initially).

Check and maintain airway. Quarter-hourly full neurological observations for 2 hours, then ½-hourly full neurological observations for 2 hours are performed. These are then reduced as directed by medical staff as the patient's condition stabilizes; often 2-hourly overnight and then 4-hourly the next day.

A wash is appreciated by the patient, and he can put on his own night clothes.

Once nausea is controlled, oral fluids (water at first) may be commenced. A flexistraw is useful. A light diet may commence on the evening of the investigation — help may be required as the patient will be lying flat.

The intravenous infusion is discontinued when the patient's condition is stable, he is tolerating adequate oral fluids and he has passed urine.

As the patient has had a general anaesthetic and may have a headache, it may be advisable not to encourage visitors on the day of the test. If the patient is very anxious, however, a sensible relative may be reasuring, since the patient may have thought he was 'about to lose his head'.

NOTES:

1 Raised intracranial pressure is always present immediately postinvestigation, but it should resolve slowly. If it does not, or shows signs of increasing at any time, or any other abnormality occurs in the neurological observations, it must be reported immediately to trained staff.

2 This procedure is being superceded by newer techniques, e.g. brain scan and ultrasound, and so may rarely be carried out.

When are the results available and what might they be?

Results may not be available for 2 days or until the radiologist's report is received. Possible findings include:

1   Congenital abnormalities

2   Tumours

3   Hydrocephalus.

Contraindications for AEG

AEG is not performed when intracranial pressure is raised.

Can complications occur?

Severe nausea and headache are not uncommon, so analgesia and antiemetics should be administered, as required, to control these. Meningitis is rare and is due to faulty lumbar puncture technique.

6.2.   Cerebral angiogram

What is a cerebral angiogram?

Cerebral angiography involves insertion of a fine catheter through the femoral or brachial artery, threading it up the aorta to the aortic arch and then into either the carotid or vertebral artery, depending on the suspected area of abnormality. A radio-opaque dye is then injected through the catheter and a series of X-ray films taken very quickly to show the cerebral blood flow. It is possible to inject directly into carotid or vertebral arteries and this approach is used in some centres.

Why is a cerebral angiogram performed?

An angiogram is indicated when previous neurological investigation or history of symptoms indicate impairment of cerebral blood flow. Such indications would be unexplained loss of consciousness, vertigo attacks, severe headaches or parasthesia. After investigation diagnosis can be made of aneurysms, angiomas, occlusion of vessels and space-occupying lesions shown by alteration in vessel pattern.

Where is the cerebral angiogram performed and what preparation is necessary?

The patient is admitted 1–2 days prior to the investigation so that full assessment for suitability for general anaesthesia can be carried out. Baseline observations should be taken of temperature, pulse and respiration, and full neurological observations may also be required. A full explanation is given both to the patient and relatives, as complications can arise from this procedure, and the consent form signed. On the evening before the test a groin shave is performed to ensure a hair-free area and reduce the potential risk of infection when a femoral approach is used. The patient is prepared as for a general anaesthetic and a nurse should accompany the patient to the X-ray department where the test takes place, and remain until the patient is anaesthetized. Occasionally the investigation may be carried out under local anaesthesia, so it is even more important to explain exactly what will be happening to the patient.

The patient should be aware that there will be a number of people in the X-ray room, at least two doctors, two nurses and two radiographers. There may be some delay while all the staff are preparing the equipment. The patient is helped onto the table and some plain skull X-rays may be taken to check the position of the patient on the table.

How is the cerebral angiogram performed?

Once the patient is anaesthetized the catheter with a guidewire is introduced and threaded through the arteries under constant screening. Once the correct vessels have been reached the guidewire is removed and a small amount of dye introduced to check that the patient has no allergic reaction. If there is no reaction to the dye, the full amount is injected and a number of films taken in rapid succession to trace the passage of the dye. The duration of the test varies from 40 min to 3 hours, depending on the number and position of vessels that need visualizing, but it is usually 1–2 hours in length.

What happens after the cerebral angiogram?

Once the catheter has been removed continuous pressure must be kept onto the puncture site for at least 20 min to lessen the risk of haemorrhage. Patients vary in the time they take to come round after anaesthetic. The patient is transferred to the trolley while still asleep. According to hospital policy the patient may stay in the X-ray room until fully awake or be transferred immediately back to the ward.

Full neurological observations must be carried out every ¼-hour for 2 hours, then ½-hourly for 2 hours, being reduced at the discretion of trained staff, but usually remaining 2-hourly during the night and 4-hourly by the next morning for the following 48 hours. Nurses are particularly looking for:

1   Raised intracranial pressure, i.e., raised blood pressure and lowered pulse rate, possibly indicating cerebral haemorrhage.

2   Signs of systemic haemorrhage indicated by a lowered blood pressure and raised pulse rate.

For this reason it is vital that the nurse knows the normal levels of pulse and blood pressure of her individual patient so that abnormalities can be detected. Every time the observations are recorded the nurse must also inspect the puncture site for indications of haemorrhage, i.e., fresh blood or increasing size of haematoma. Most patients have a haematoma, but must be told that if they notice it increasing in size or starting to bleed they must call a nurse immediately.

The patient must lay flat for 24 hours and keep his arm or leg where the puncture site is as still as possible to reduce the risk of haemorrhage. Lying flat also reduces the risk of headache and prescribed analgesia must be given. As soon as the patient is awake and not nauseated he may drink, and he may eat the following day, help being needed as he will be lying flat. He will appreciate a wash and a change of night attire.

The patient will be drowsy after this investigation so visitors are not advisable on the day of the test, but if the patient is very anxious a sensible relative may be reassuring to the patient.

When are the results available and what might they be?

The results will not be available for a few days as they have to be seen and reported on by the radiologist and then the results communicated to the patient's medical team. Possible findings include:

1   Aneurysms.
2   Angiomas.
3   Vessel occlusion.
4   Space-occupying lesions.

Contraindications for a cerebral angiogram

There are no contraindications.

Can complications occur?

Possible complications could include the following:

1   Risk of haemorrhage:
    a. From site in groin or elbow where catheter was removed so this must be inspected every time the observations are done.
    b. Internal — there is always a slight risk of haemorrhage due to the puncture of vessels so again accurate observations are vital.

c. Cerebral — because of the increased pressure within the brain where the dye is introduced and observations indicating raised blood pressure and lowered pulse rate would indicate this.

2 Thrombi and emboli can also occur because plaques can be dislodged from the linings of arteries by the catheter, but these are rare resulting in a cerebrovascular accident.

3 Reactions to the dye can occur, but are prevented by the use of a test dose.

Patients' comments

'More frightened about general anaesthetic than the investigation, and even the general anaesthetic is nothing to worry about — in fact the injection I was given on the ward before the investigation was a marvellous feeling — my husband said that he had never seen me looking so drunk! I was given another injection in my hand and went straight off to sleep. I was told the results the following day.'

'I thought I would feel awful after the investigation, but had no sickness afterwards and felt fine. When I woke up I had a beautiful bruise in my groin where the dye had been injected, but there was no discomfort.'

'I understood about the investigation and this made me not worry. Some dye is injected into an artery by your neck or in your groin and then detailed colour X-rays are taken to show the blood vessels to the brain very clearly. Marvellous investigation, so clever, and you are asleep so it is not frightening.'

6.3.   Electroencephalogram (EEG)

What is an electroencephalogram (EEG)?

An electroencephalogram is a measurement of the electrical activity that occurs in the brain. Nerve impulses are electrical discharges and detection and recording of these will give indication to the electrical patterns within the brain — so-called 'brainwaves'. The measurements are made by numerous electrical pads that are placed on the scalp always in a set pattern. The test can be done as an outpatient and takes $1/2$–3 hours, depending on the exact technique used.

Why is an EEG performed?

Electroencephalography may be used in the differential diagnosis of the following conditions:

1   Epilepsy and other fits.

2   Cerebral lesions.

3   Vertigo attacks.

4   Loss of consciousness.

5   Headaches and flashing lights.

6   To indicate the level of confusion in toxic states caused by trauma and jaundice.

7   To identify an organic cause for mental illness.

8   To confirm brain death.

From the graph of the electrical activity in the brain normal and abnormal patterns may be identified and, depending on their nature and the leads that they are associated with, differential diagnosis may be possible.

Where is the EEG performed and what preparation is necessary?

The technique is entirely noninvasive and painless. It is performed in an EEG department. The patient is asked to wash his hair the night before the test as grease reduces the contact between scalp and electrodes. For the same reason he is asked not to apply hair lacquer or oil. It is advisable to warn him that his hair may need washing after the test as contact jelly is used which may leave the hair sticky. If the patient has been taking benzodiazepine night sedation, i.e., Mogadon or Dalmaine, he may be asked not to take it on the night before the test as it can induce abnormal activity which would alter vital patterns. Sometimes a sleep deprivation test is carried out. The patient will be asked to stay awake for the night previous to the investigation. In this case the test is best done in the afternoon after the sleepless night when the patient is feeling the effect of his lack of sleep most. This is because lack of sleep will make the patient more likely to be drowsy and drift off to sleep while the electroencephalogram is being performed. A sleep recording is often desirable as the drowsy state is said to 'activate' the record, i.e., enhance any abnormalities. Another technique of obtaining a sleeping trace is the oral administration of quinalbarbitone (Seconal), 20 mg, which will cause the patient to be drowsy, but this also means that he will remain drowsy when the test is over and he may have to go home. For this reason the sleep deprivation method is preferable. Chlorpromazine, either orally or by intramuscular injection, can be used to sedate uncooperative patients. It is vital that the patient has eaten a normal diet prior to the test as hypoglycaemia can alter otherwise normal patterns. If hypoglycaemia is suspected by the technicians, an oral glucose drink is given and the wait for this to be absorbed prolongs the test when it could easily have been avoided.

How is the EEG performed?

When the patient goes to the test room he will probably first be asked to go to the toilet and empty his bladder so that he will feel comfortable during the test. Then he will be asked to sit in a chair while the electrodes are put in position. There are two methods of connecting electrodes. One is placing over the head a rubber cap, rather like a firm hairnet, which can be used to hold the electrode pads in position. This is used for short readings, as after about ½ hour the pressure of the pads can cause discomfort. The other method is to use smaller electrodes which are laid on the scalp, a piece of hair placed over the top and some contact gel applied so that the hair is sticky and holds the electrode in position on the scalp. This method is less uncomfortable and holds the electrodes more securely onto the scalp. Therefore it is used when sleeping recordings are made as the electrodes will not fall off if the patient turns over.

In both cases at least 23 electrode pads are applied to the scalp. Where each electrode touches the scalp, the scalp is first cleaned with methylated spirit at a parting in the hair and then a small amount of contact gel is applied. When all the electrodes are in position the patient is either settled more comfortably in an armchair or asked to lie down. When he is in a relaxed position the leads are attached to the electrodes and then to the recording machine. The lights in the room are then switched out and the patient asked to relax while the machine runs.

During the test certain techniques are commonly used to enhance abnormal brain activity. These are called 'activation techniques'. The first is hyperventilation where the patient is asked to hyperventilate for one or two periods at 3-min intervals and in some doing induces hypocapnia. This will make his feet and hands tingle if it is done properly. The other method is the use of a strobe light, which is flashed at different frequencies in a set sequence so that the frequency which induces the abnormal pattern can be easily identified.

Apart from the short periods of hyperventilation all the patient has to do during the test is lie down and try to relax. Although at first the rubber cap and electrode pads may seem very frightening, once the patient knows they are not painful and has become accustomed to the humming made by the running of the machine he will relax, and many patients drift off to sleep.

What happens after the EEG?

When the test is finished the electrodes and cap are removed. The scalp is wiped as clean as possible and the patient is free to go home. As this test is entirely noninvasive there is no aftercare or complications, making it a reliable test of choice for primary diagnosis. If sedation has been given the patient will be advised not to drive and should have a friend or relative available to take them home. Its findings are only conclusive in a few cases, e.g., petit mal epilepsy, hepatic encephalopathy or other epileptic foci, but the test will often give an indication as to whether further investigations are needed.

When are the results available and what might they be?

After the EEG tracings have been studied by the doctor in the EEG department, a report will be sent to the patient's doctor, so there may be a delay of 2–3 days before full results are known. Possible findings include:

1   Cerebral lesions.
2   Areas of abnormal brain activity.
3   Areas of tissue death.

Contraindications for an EEG.

There are no contraindications.

6.4.   Lumbar Puncture

What is a lumbar puncture?

The procedure involves the introduction of a needle under strict aseptic conditions into the lumbar subarachnoid space below the termination of the spinal cord. The cord is much shorter than the canal in which it lies, and itself only extends down to the first lumbar vertebrae. Conveniently this allows a space from which a sample of cerebrospinal fluid can be extracted without risk of damage to the spinal cord. The needle is passed through the intervertebral space between the third and fourth, or fourth and fifth lumbar vertebra. There are measurable changes that take place in the cerebrospinal fluid (CSF) so the purpose of the puncture in diagnosis is to determine the pressure of the CSF and to obtain specimens of the fluid for examination.

Why is a lumbar puncture performed?

The lumbar puncture may be performed for the following reasons:

1   To estimate CSF pressure to demonstrate any blockage of the subarachnoid pathways. Normal CSF pressure varies from 60 to 180 mm H_2O. It is also affected by pulse and blood pressure. The flexed position also increases the pressure, therefore, the manometer reading should be recorded with the patient in a relaxed position after entry of lumbar puncture needle.

2   To obtain CSF for diagnostic purposes, e.g., confirmation of a subarachnoid haemorrhage or meningitis. Normally CSF is clear and colourless. Immediately after a subarachnoid haemorrhage the CSF is blood stained. After a time it becomes xanthochromic (yellow in colour) due to the breakdown of red blood cells. If meningitis is suspected a specimen of CSF will be sent to the laboratory for estimation of cell protein, chloride and glucose content, culture of organisms and antibiotic sensitivity tests. CSF stagnating below a spinal block may be yellow in colour and will have an increased protein content.

3   CSF may be examined for the presence of pathogenic organisms, e.g., in the case of suspected secondary or tertiary syphilis.

4   Special tests may be performed on the CSF, such as the colloidal gold reaction if multiple sclerosis is suspected.

5   A lumbar puncture may be performed for diagnosis by contrast radiography. A contrast medium, such as air for outlining the ventricular system (see airencephalography, Section 6.1) or radio-opaque liquid for spinal exploration (see myelography, Section 5.2).

6   After surgery a lumbar puncture is sometimes performed as a palliative measure to relieve hydrocephalus. Since this is an extremely dangerous procedure it may only be performed when medical treatment has been ineffective.

7   A lumbar puncture can be used as a way of introducing drugs in the case of cerebral infection where drugs given by other routes do not cross the blood brain barrier.

Where is the lumbar puncture performed and what preparations are necessary?

A full explanation of the procedure is given to the patient, and, if required by local policy, a consent form is signed. Questions are encouraged and answered. There are no dietary restrictions for this procedure. Preparation may include shaving the lumbar region. Scrupulous hygiene of the area is essential. Either a bath or blanket bath is given and a clean gown and bed linen are provided. The bladder should be emptied to enable the patient to relax. Privacy and dignity should be ensured.

The most important factor in achieving a successful lumbar puncture is the correct positioning of the patient and his cooperation should always be gained. The patient is normally asked to lie on his left side with his back right up against the edge of the bed. The knees should be drawn up and the head and trunk flexed to widen the interspinous spaces, so that the doctor can more easily insert the needle. This position may be difficult to achieve if the patient has a spinal or muscular condition which inhibits flexion of the spine. The nurse helps by supporting the patient behind the neck and knees and by helping the patient to keep still. Asking the patient to breathe deeply is a useful distraction to help him relax. The patient must be told not to move or cough (cough linctus may be required) and to ask the nurse if he requires to move or needs anything.

The actual procedure, which is performed by a senior doctor, will take not more than 10 min, with, possibly, a further 10 min preparation and positioning time.

How is the lumbar puncture performed?

Strict aseptic technique is necessary to prevent the introduction of infection into the spinal cord. Masks should be worn. After thoroughly cleaning the area with iodine (or antiseptic of choice) the doctor then usually administers a local anaesthetic (2% lignocaine — 5 ml ampoule is adequate) to the area to minimize discomfort. The patient may experience an initial stinging sensation when the local anaesthetic is injected, then the only pain should be that of pressure as the doctor inserts the larger lumbar puncture needle. By attaching a manometer to the needle the doctor will measure the pressure. He may wish to do the Queckenstedt's test to test the patency of the CSF pathway. The nurse may be asked to apply manual pressure to one or both jugular veins whilst the CSF pressure is recorded on the manometer. This is a potentially dangerous manoeuvre if both veins are compressed simultaneously as it can result in transtentorial or tonsillar herniation. If there is a thrombosis of a jugular vein or obstruction in the CSF pathway, as by a spinal tumour, the level in the manometer may not rise, or do so slowly, and fail to fall when the pressure is released.

CSF, 8–10 ml, is collected in three labelled specimen bottles — numbered 1, 2 and 3. The reason for this is that specimen 1 is often contaminated with blood from the insertion of the needle and, therefore, can be ignored. Blood found in specimen 2 or 3 is of diagnostic significance and may confirm a suspected subarachnoid or cerebrovascular haemorrhage. These laboratory tests may take up to 1 week to complete. The needle is withdrawn and a collodion occlusive dressing is applied.

What happens after the lumbar puncture?

The patient is made comfortable with one pillow for 6–12 hours. Neurological observations may be requested. The site should be checked for leakage. The patient should be encouraged to eat and drink. The body will replace the CSF within 2 days.

When are the results available and what might they be?

The results from the pathology department may take up to 1 week to be reported. Possible findings include:

1   Raised intracranial pressure.

2   Infection, e.g., meningitis.

3   Subarachnoid haemorrhage.

Contraindications for a lumbar puncture

There are certain contraindications:

1   If raised intracranial pressure is suspected, or if a stroke patient's level of consciousness is lowered, then it is dangerous to perform a lumbar puncture.

2   If there is a high level of meningeal infection or skin sepsis.

3   If there is suspected cord compression. In many isolated spinal cord lesions it is impossible to distinguish an intrinsic lesion (e.g., multiple sclerosis) from extrinsic compression. Myelography with CSF examination is then necessary rather than a separate lumbar puncture.

Can complications occur?

Complications may include the following:

1   The patient may complain of headache after the procedure. This is normally attributed either to the removal of CSF during the test or to later leakage of the fluid into the tissues. The headache is normally relieved by having the patient remain in a horizontal position for 6–12 hours. An icebag can be applied to the head and a mild analgesic may be prescribed. If the headache persists or becomes increasingly severe the doctor should be contacted immediately.

2   If signs of an increase in intracranial pressure become evident the patient's level of consciousness, pulse, respiration, blood pressure and papillary reactions are observed and recorded every 30 min for the first 2 hours, and then every hour for the next 12 hours. Any adverse change is reported to the doctor immediately.

3   If, during the test, the needle is not introduced in the midline it may contact one of the dorsal nerve roots and cause pain down one leg. This can be rectified immediately by removing the needle and the patient is reassured that no damage has been done.

4   The procedure is considerably more difficult to carry out successfully if the patient is obese as the vertebrae will be much more difficult to detect.

5   Pressure coning — this can occur if some degree of raised intracranial pressure was present prior to the lumbar puncture. Normally this is a contraindication for this investigation. Pressure coning is herniation of downward movement of the cerebellar tonsils so that they impact within the foramen magnum thus compressing the medulla.

6   Backache is not uncommon.

Further Reading

Chapman S and Nakielny R (1981) Guide to Radiological Procedures, Baillière Tindall

MacLeod J (editor) (1981) Davidson's Principles and Practice of Medicine, 13th edition, Churchill Livingstone

Scott D (1976) Understanding the EEG, Duckworth

Shetler M (1981) Spinal and peritoneal taps when quick action counts, Registered Nurse 44: 50–53

Sutton D (1977) Radiology for Medical Students, 3rd edition, Churchill Livingstone

Weir J and Abrahams P (1978) Atlas of Radiological Anatomy, Pitman Medical

Zwanenburg D and Adams C (1979) Neurosurgical Nursing Care, Faber & Faber

CHAPTER 7

INVESTIGATIONS ASSOCIATED WITH THE RESPIRATORY SYSTEM

The respiratory tract includes the nasal passages, pharynx, larynx, trachea, main bronchi and lungs and associated pleura.

Oxygen is essential to life, so any diminution of the supply to the vital organs like the brain, heart and kidneys will rapidly lead to altered function or death.

Breathlessness is always distressing and frightening to both the patient and his relatives. Investigations which might cause further respiratory embarrassment must therefore be carefully explained and adequate support given.

7.1. Bronchography

What is a bronchogram?

Bronchography is a special X-ray investigation of the lungs. It involves the introduction of an iodized oil, which is radio-opaque, into the bronchi, so that X-ray films can be taken to give a complete outline of each bronchial tree.

Why is a bronchogram performed?

The main indication for performing a bronchogram is for the assessment of bronchiectasis. Bronchography is rarely used to demonstrate other abnormalities of the bronchi as the major bronchi are much better seen under direct vision, i.e., bronchoscopy. It also provides useful additional information in certain respiratory disease when trying to establish a diagnosis.

Where is a bronchogram performed and what preparation is necessary?

The patient should be prepared psychologically by the nurse giving a simple comprehensive explanation of the examination and answering any

97

questions. A consent form may be required to be signed. Good preparation includes some or all of the following points, although there is variation between different departments and hospitals.

1   For 3 days prior to the examination the patient should take 600 mg potassium iodine three times daily as it increases expectoration. Thus accumulation of secretions in the bronchi are removed during coughing, ensuring that when the contrast agent is introduced into the bronchial tree a better filling is obtained. It also indicates whether the patient has a sensitivity to iodine.

2   For 3 days prior to the examination the bronchial tree is cleared of secretions as far as possible by postural coughing. Postural drainage consists of tipping the patient into various positions so that gravity will encourage accumulated mucus to drain from the lungs.

3   The patient should have a light diet on the day of the examination, but should have nothing by mouth for at least 4 hours prior to bronchography. This is to prevent inhalation of vomit during the procedure.

4   Finally atropine may be given by subcutaneous injection ½ hour before bronchography is performed to reduce bronchial secretions.

5   The patient should don an open-backed gown immediately before the examination, and jewellery, glasses and false teeth should be removed.

How is the bronchogram performed?

Bronchography takes place in the X-ray department — the patient will be sent for about 10 min before the examination is due to take place. There are currently two main methods of introducing the contrast agent into the trachea:

1   Via a pernasal endotracheal catheter.

2   Via a catheter introduced percutaneously through the cricothyroid membrane.

Bronchography may be performed under local anaesthesia or general anaesthesia. It is very important that the full cooperation of the patient is obtained for the bronchography to be successfully completed. For this reason very nervous patients and children under the age of 7 are usually examined under general anaesthesia. The patient lies supine on the X-ray table with a small pillow under his shoulders with his head and neck extended. A premedication is given intramuscularly — pethidine and scopolamine are the most common agents used. The whole examination takes between 30 and 60 min.

During pernasal endotracheal intubation the patient is asked to sniff a lignocaine solution through the more patent nostril and the rest of the airway is anaesthetized, either by the patient gargling lignocaine solution or by the use of a laryngeal spray. The doctor attempts to pass the catheter blind by standing behind a seated patient and passing the catheter along the floor of the nasal passages. By compressing the patient's larynx lightly against the cervical spine the passage of the catheter is encouraged through the vocal cords. To confirm the position of the catheter the patient is asked to phonate — only a whisper or shrill note will be heard. If difficulty is encountered the patient is asked to lie supine on the table and a laryngoscope is used. During the cricothyroid method the skin over the cricothyroid membrane is cleaned and lignocaine is injected into the tissues down to the membrane to obtain local anaesthesia. This will cause the patient to cough. A needle is then introduced through the membrane and a catheter guided through the needle into the trachea. The catheter is then secured in place with strapping (check the patient is not allergic to strapping). The contrast medium, e.g., dionosic oily 60%, is introduced into the catheter with the patient lying on the side to be examined; 1 ml of oil is used for each year of the patient's life, up to a maximum of 12 ml. The patient is then rolled forwards to fill the middle lobe and anterior segments of the upper and lower lobes and backwards to fill the apical lower bronchus and posterior segments of the upper and lower lobes. The patient is securely strapped to the table which is then briefly tilted head downwards to fill the apical segment of the upper lobe.

Once filling of the bronchial tree is complete, films are taken with the table level. The left side is filled in the same manner, but more slowly as there is a tendency to cough more when oil is present in the opposite bronchial tree. One side is visualized at a time as this reduces the risk of side-effects.

Dionosil is the medium most commonly used as it is rapidly absorbed and excreted by the kidneys and consequently does not remain in the lungs.

What happens after the bronchogram?

The patient will certainly want to remain in bed for a few hours following a bronchography as it is very tiring and can be quite distressing to the patient.

The patient should not take anything by mouth for at least 3 hours after the bronchography until the tracheal anaesthetic has worn off. The patient should be clearly warned of the danger of food or drink 'going the wrong way'. Observations of pulse and respiration should be performed ½-hourly for 2 hours, to observe for respiratory embarrassment, and reduced when stable.

Finally, the patient should receive extensive physiotherapy to enable him to expectorate any oil left in the lungs and any secretions. A mouth wash and wash may be appreciated.

When are the results available and what might they be?

The results should be available in 2–3 days after the radiologist has reported on the X-rays taken. Possible findings include:

1   The extent of bronchiectasis.
2   Neoplasms.

Contraindications for a bronchogram

This procedure is unlikely to be performed on a patient with severe respiratory embarrassment.

Can complications occur?

Rarely, the patient may have an adverse reaction to the contrast medium or the patient may suffer respiratory impairment or arrest.

7.2.   Bronchoscopy (fibreoptic)

What is a bronchoscopy?

Bronchoscopy is a procedure for direct visual assessment of patency, confirmation of obstruction by foreign bodies or pathological involvement of the respiratory tract.

It is not only a diagnostic procedure, but allows access to the lower reaches of the trachea and main bronchial tubes for removal of a foreign body or for biopsy to be taken.

What is a bronchoscope?

The fibreoptic bronchoscope is a hollow tube, black in colour, and 35 cm long (just over 14 in). The fibreoptic light is encased within the bronchoscope and it allows good illumination. There is also a small channel which is connected to suction. The tip of the bronchoscope can be moved in various directions by the operator and an eyepiece at the other end allows direct vision of the respiratory passages.

Why is a bronchoscopy performed?

Possible reasons for carrying out this procedure are as follows:

1   To remove a foreign body.
2   To facilitate free air passage, e.g., removal of a mucous plug.
3   To obtain a biopsy from the bronchi or a sample of bronchial secretions.
4   To observe the air passages for signs of disease and carcinoma.
5   To diagnose abnormalities or obstruction.

Where is the bronchoscopy performed and what preparation is necessary?

This investigation can be carried out either as an inpatient or an outpatient provided adequate preparation is given.

Bronchoscopy is ususally performed in a laboratory away from the ward area by a doctor who specializes in diseases of the respiratory system.

The procedure should be explained and questions encouraged and answered. In most hospitals a consent form must be signed by the patient. The patient should be told that he will have to breathe through his mouth throughout the investigation as the bronchoscope is passed down through the nostril. The patient should have nothing by mouth for at least 4 hours prior to the investigation. Mouth care and toilet can be offered to the patient. Dentures, braces and plates should be removed as the patient will be drowsy and it is easier to maintain a clear airway without these. Glasses and contact lenses should also be removed as they get in the way of the bronchoscope. The patient is asked to rest in a semiupright position on a couch. In most cases the patient is asked to keep as still as possible during the investigation. He should be warned that his sputum may be bloodstained for a few hours or days after the investigation if the doctor has taken a biopsy. If bleeding continues for a long period or is excessive, the doctor should be notified. The patient's notes, X-rays and charts usually accompany him to the investigation, as should a ward nurse.

How is the bronchoscopy performed?

The patient is made comfortable in a suitable position, usually semirecumbent or lying down. A needle suitable for giving intermittent intravenous drugs is inserted into a vein in the arm. A premedication is then given intravenously to sedate the patient and also limit bronchial secretions. In most cases the sedation prescribed is a respiratory depressant.

The patient's nostril is anaesthetized with a topical local anaesthetic such as lignocaine. The taste may not be very pleasant for the patient and may cause some discomfort. The bronchoscope is then passed down via the nose, through the larynx into the trachea, until the two main bronchi are visualized, then each main bronchus is explored. A biopsy of a tumour or a group of cells can be taken with the biopsy forceps, which are passed down the bronchoscope. Once the biopsy has been taken bleeding occurs which will occlude vision. A 'brush' specimen or a light abrasion of a lesion can be taken, which is mounted on a glass slide. Bronchial secretions are collected in a small trap and this can be sent to the laboratory to screen for malignant cells.

If a biopsy is taken during the procedure, blood loss is usually minimal, but the patient may find he has bloodstained sputum for severals hours or days. When the doctor has finished the examination and all specimens have been collected the bronchoscope is removed. The patient is gently aroused with the news that the examination has finished and he is left 5 or 10 min to recover. The intravenous cannula can then be removed from the arm before the patient is helped to a wheelchair. The patient is then taken to a recovery area, which may be in the laboratory or he may return to his ward where he will be allowed to sleep off the effects of the drugs given.

Rigid tubular bronchoscopes may still be in use in certain areas and these are illuminated with a small electric lamp. When using this type of bronchoscope the patient is placed in a supine position with the head downwards so that the larynx and trachea are in a straight line. Patients can also sit upright, though this is not the safest position.

What happens after the bronchoscopy?

Position the patient on his left side in bed and check that his airway is free from any secretions. Let the patient rest and/or sleep off the effects of the drugs. Suction and oxygen equipment should be available. Carry out specific orders given by the doctor with regard to specific care or keep the patient 'nil by mouth' for 3–4 hours until the swallow reflex returns. Offer oral hygiene to the patient when he wakes up. Encourage the patient to cough and expectorate so that any mucus can be cleared from the bronchi.

The patient should remain in bed until he is fully awake and should be supervised, if necessary, when he first gets out of bed.

If a biopsy has been taken during bronchoscopy ½-hourly recordings of pulse and blood pressure should be taken until the patient's condition is satisfactory. Observe the patient for any complications and contact the doctor if necessary. When the swallow reflex returns sips of water may be given. If this is tolerated well, the patient may eat and drink as he wishes. Simple linctus can usually be given to the patient as prescribed if he has a sore throat. Smoking shortly after a bronchoscopy is not advisable as it can irritate the bronchial lining. If the patient does haemorrhage following a biopsy his pulse will most probably increase and his blood pressure decrease. He will have an irritating cough and is likely to have bloodstained mucus or sputum. Keep the patient in bed and keep him calm. Contact the doctor and observe the colour of the patient while recording observations of pulse and blood pressure.

An outpatient can usually be discharged once he is fully awake and the doctor is satisfied with his condition. It is advisable for a relative or friend to accompany the patient home.

When are the results available and what might they be?

The initial results following a bronchoscopy are available to the patient as soon as the doctor visits the patient following the procedure. Results from specimens of mucus or a biopsy will take several days to return from the laboratory. The length of stay in hospital will depend upon the reason for the bronchoscopy.

Possible results are:

1   Carcinoma.

2   Obstruction by, for example, pin, button, dentures, fish bone.

3   Pulmonary abscess.

4   Tuberculosis.

5   Bronchiectasis.

Contraindications for a bronchoscopy

1   Upper respiratory tract infection.

2   Recent meal.

3   Laryngeal abnormalities.

Can complications occur?

Possible complications arising from this procedure could include:

1   Dyspnoea.

2   Oedema of glottis.

3   Loss of gag reflex and inhalation of secretions.

4   Spasm of larynx.

5   Haemorrhage following a biopsy.

6   Hoarseness, or sore throat.

7   Respiratory arrest.

Patients' comments

'It was an investigation to look at my lungs and wind pipes. Very clever. I was asleep all of the time, but it would have been interesting to watch I am sure!'

'I had nothing to eat or drink for 6 hours before the investigation. I had my injection on the ward, which made me feel very sleepy. I wasn't worried because it was fully explained and it is nothing to be frightened about. I knew what it was for and what happened.'

'I know tubes went down my throat for my doctor to see inside my pipes. When I woke up my mouth was very dry, but I had no soreness. I was given sips of water, but didn't eat or drink for several hours until my throat felt better.'

7.3.   Chest Aspiration

What is a chest aspiration?

Removal of fluid or air from pleural space by means of a needle introduced through an intercostal space.

Why is a chest aspiration performed?

Possible reasons for carrying out this procedure could be as follows:

1   For diagnostic purposes, especially when malignant disease is suspected. A specimen of pleural fluid is collected and sent to the laboratory.

2   Therapeutically to relieve symptoms, e.g., dyspnoea:
   a. In a pleural effusion the fluid is aspirated.
   b. In a case of emphysema or a haemothorax.
   c. In pneumothorax the procedure is followed and a chest drain introduced.
   d. To instil a drug into the pleural cavity, e.g., a cytotoxic drug.

Where is the chest aspiration performed and what preparation is necessary?

Chest aspiration is usually performed in the ward. Full explanation should be given to the patient, questions encouraged and answered. A chest X-ray should be taken prior to the investigation and this should be available for the doctor to see. If the skin surface is hairy it should be shaved from midaxilla to the centre of the back covering the affected lung area. A dressing trolley should be prepared following the hospital procedure with all the requirements needed for a chest aspiration. If the patient has a cough, simple linctus can be given as prescribed. The patient must tell the doctor if he wishes to cough during the procedure. The patient should empty his bladder prior to the procedure so that he is comfortable.

Make the patient comfortable sitting on the end of the bed. His arms should be folded on a pillow placed on a bed table. The patient should be able to lean forwards so that the ribs and scapulae are retracted away from the middle. If the patient is unable to sit upright, he can lean his unaffected side on the bed. His arm will be supported above his head. Provide a warm blanket for the patient and ensure adequate privacy. If possible stand by the patient's head to help him maintain his position and give him support throughout the procedure. A second nurse can assist the doctor with the procedure. Patients are allowed to eat and drink normally before this investigation. The patient is awake and though this procedure should not be painful if local anaesthetic is used correctly the patient will feel a small prick in the skin and perhaps a feeling of pressure. Clear instructions must be given to the patient about the need to regulate his breathing pattern, as requested by the doctor, during this procedure.

How is the chest aspiration performed?

The chest X-ray is usually viewed by the doctor and he will often listen to breath sounds prior to aspirating the fluid. These sounds are reduced over the effusion area. With the patient in the correct position the skin is cleaned with an antiseptic solution. The ribs are palpated and the chest wall percussed. Over the effusion a stony dull note is produced compared to a resonant normal side. The skin is anaesthetized with local anaesthetic, usually lignocaine. The 50 ml syringe and aspiration needle are assembled together and the needle is inserted above the rib in the required site. Intercostal vessels and nerves run along the lower edge of the rib so a needle aimed for the pleural space should be passed above the rib to avoid these structures. The needle is pushed carefully into the chest.

'Sucking back' is carried out to make sure the needle is not within a vein. When the pleura is felt the needle is pushed through the pleura and the resistance disappears, fluid may now be aspirated from the pleural space. To prevent the needle slipping further in and causing damage to the lung a pair of Spencer Wells forceps are clipped onto the needle. When the syringe is full of fluid the tap is turned and the fluid is drained into the sterile jug. The maximum amount of fluid aspirated at any one time is 500 ml because cardiac complications can occur when the mediastinum swings back into its usual position. During the procedure observe the patient's condition, his degree of pain and respiratory function. The procedure can be quite exhausting and may take ¾ hour or longer, depending how easily the fluid or air can be removed.

When all the fluid has been removed the needle is withdrawn and the site is covered with an occlusive dressing, i.e., plastic spray dressing and a piece of gauze.

What happens after the chest aspiration?

Patients should be encouraged to stay in bed for at least 1 hour after the procedure, lying on the unaffected side. Observe the pulse, blood pressure, respirations ½-hourly for at least 2 to 3 hours, or until the patient's condition is satisfactory. Four-hourly temperature and pulse are continued for 2 days. Observe the dressing for haemorrhage or fluid loss every ½ hour for 2–3 hours following the procedure. Observe for any difficulty in breathing, haemoptysis, colour or any complications and contact the doctor if necessary. Give regular analgesia as prescribed, if required. Give the patient a bell.

Record on the fluid balance chart the type of fluid and the volume aspirated. Label the specimen bottles and send them with the completed microbiology and cytology forms to the laboratory. Record in the nursing kardex the appropriate information. A repeat X-ray will be taken. Patients can eat and drink after this investigation. Visitors are permitted as long as the patient's condition is satisfactory.

When are the results available and what might they be?

If a chest aspiration is performed to relieve symptoms from a pleural effusion, the patient should appreciate the results almost immediately, as breathing becomes easier. If specimens of pleural fluid have been sent for cytology and microbiology investigations, the results will be received after 2–3 days. Possible results/findings include:

1   Haemothorax following trauma.

2   Chylothorax (accumulation of lymph in the pleural cavity) following damage to the thoracic duct.

3   Infection such as pleurisy following a bacterial pneumonia or pulmonary tuberculosis.

4   Malignant disease which has involved the pleura.

Contraindications for a chest aspiration

1   A very confused, uncooperative patient.

2   A patient with a persistent, uncontrollable cough for whom sedation is inappropriate

Can complications occur?

Possible complications include:

1   Dyspnoea.

2   Faintness.

3   Severe pain.

4   Pneumothorax — the introduction of air through the aspiration hole following the procedure.

5   Cardiac complications — arrhythmias as the displaced mediastinum swings back into position.

6   Haemothorax — inadvertent puncture of the lung surface with subsequent bleeding.

7   Surgical emphysema — an escape of air from the pleural space into the subcutaneous tissues.

8   Acute pulmonary oedema.

9   Haemoptysis — following trauma to the lung.

Patients' comments

'It was uncomfortable, but worth it as I can now breathe more easily.'

'I was tired when they finished, but it did help my breathing.'

7.4.   Lung Function Tests

The main function of the respiratory system is to oxygenate the blood flowing through the pulmonary capillaries and remove excess carbon dioxide, thus maintaining the arterial gases at pressures within a narrow physiological range.

What are lung function tests?

Lung function tests are a method of assessing the efficiency of the respiratory system, particularly with respect to ventilation, i.e., the movement of air into and out of the lungs.

Why are lung function tests performed?

Lung function tests play little part in the diagnosis of disease, but they do allow assessment of the nature and extent of pulmonary involvement in disease processes such as sarcoidosis, cough disorders, chronic bronchitis and emphysema.

Lung function tests allow the assessment of the effects of treatment, e.g., steroid treatment in sarcoidosis, can be useful as an early warning sign of deterioration in an asthmatic patient, i.e., a fall in the peak flow rate and can be used to assess the fitness of a patient for anaesthesia and surgery. Lung function tests provide a guide as to the extent of physiotherapy required postoperatively. The forced expectoratory volume demonstrates the patient's ability to cough up secretions and, for the purpose of thoracic surgery, they indicate whether the remaining lung tissue will be capable of maintaining efficient respiration.

Lung function tests can be used to detect the respiratory consequences of skeletal disorders, such as ankylosing spondilitis, and in the detection and management of industrial diseases, e.g., asbestosis and allergic alcolitis.

Chest diseases are characterized by a decreased ablity to move air in and out of the lungs freely. Measurements of lung volumes shows the volume of gas moved in and out of the lungs during quiet and forced respiration and how easily the volume of air is moved. They also show the amount of air in the respiratory passages and alveoli at different stages of breathing.

Obstructive defects, e.g., chronic bronchitis and emphysema increase the resistance to air flow in small airways, therefore, slowing the rate of expiration, although the vital capacity remains the same. Pulmonary fibrotic changes, on the other hand, give rise to stiff lungs which contract sharply after full inspiration and cause a high-speed expiration, although the vital capacity is reduced.

Where are lung function tests performed and what preparation is necessary?

The patient is usually required to go to a lung function laboratory but some tests may be performed on the ward or in the outpatients department where portable apparatus, such as a vitalograph, may be available. There is no pre- or postinvestigative preparation for a patient undergoing lung function tests.

How are lung function tests performed?

Forced vital capacity and forced expiratory volume   Forced vital capacity (FVC) and forced expiratory volume (FEV) in 1 second are the two most common measurements made. The patient is asked to inspire maximally and breathe out into a spirometer as fast and as much as he can. The volume of expired air delivered in the first second is the FEV and the total volume is the FVC. By dividing the FEV_1 by the FVC and multiplying by 100 the FEV percentage is obtained. The age, sex and height of the patient is taken into consideration when interpreting the results.

The normal average volumes are as follows:

FEV_1: 3.0 litres,

FVC: 4.0 litres,

FEV %: 75%.

The vitalograph is a form of spirometer and is used to measure the FEV_1 and the FVC.

Sometimes bronchodilators will be given as an inhalation and the measurements repeated to assess their effects.

Peak expiratory flow   Peak expiratory flow rate is measured on a Wrights peak flow meter and is a similar indicator to FEV_1. A Wrights peak flow meter consists of a large calibrated dial with a mouthpiece. (More modern peak flow meters are tube-shaped with the calibrations along the side of the tube.) The patient is asked to inspire maximally and exhale into the peak flow meter as fast and as much as he can. The dial moves to read off the rate of air flow during forced expiration in litres per minute. To ensure accuracy the subject is asked to do this three times and the average peak flow rate is recorded. Again age, sex and height are taken into consideration — the average normal value is 416–650 l/min.

Residual volume   The residual volume is the amount of air left in the lungs following a forced expiration and amounts to 1–1.5 l. This can never be expelled from the lungs. It can be measured using the helium dilution method. Helium is a light inert gas which can be breathed without harmful effect. Helium is readily detected and as it can be breathed in and out without being absorbed at normal atmospheric pressure it can be used to measure residual volume. The patient sits upright and breathes normally through a tube into the apparatus for 10 min. The gas mixture of 21% oxygen and a known amount of helium is respired and analysed at the end of the test. Helium mixes with the residual air normally present within the lungs and residual air dilutes the helium by an amount exactly related to the air volume. After final gas analysis a simple calculation shows the residual volume.

Diffusing capacity   Measurement of diffusing capacity of the lungs assesses the extent of respiratory impairment. The patient is asked to breathe in a special gas mixture containing a small amount of carbon monoxide, hold it for 10 s and then breathe out. During expiration a sample of the expired air is taken and analysed for traces of carbon monoxide. Carbon monoxide combines readily with haemoglobin and if gaseous exchange is good the carbon monoxide will be taken up. If gaseous exchange is poor less carbon monoxide will be taken up and there will be a greater concentration in the expired air. Comparison shows transfer ability of patient's respiratory system.

Blood gas analysis   Blood gas analysis is conveniently put under the heading of lung function tests as it gives an indication of the efficiency of the lungs in transferring oxygen and carbon dioxide between the alveolar air and the blood. The patient is made comfortable. The femoral, brachial or radial arteries may be used. Using a 2–5 ml syringe containing a small amount of low concentration heparin, i.e., 1000 units/ml, the artery is punctured and a sample of blood taken. The analysis is carried out immediately. Meanwhile pressure is applied to the punctured artery for at least 3 min to prevent the formation of a haematoma. The report on blood gas analysis should state the partial pressures of oxygen ($P\text{O}_2$), carbon dioxide ($P\text{CO}_2$), the pH of the blood and the standard bicarbonate. The normal values are as follows:

$P\text{O}_2 = 11.3–14.0 \text{ kPa (100 mmHg)}$

$P\text{CO}_2 = 4.7–6.0 \text{ kPa (40 mmHg)}$

$\text{pH} = 7.4$

Standard bicarbonate = 26 mmol/l

When are the results available and what might they be?

The results are available as soon as they have been analysed, usually within 24 hours, and will indicate the extent of pulmonary disease.

Contraindications for lung function tests

There are no contraindications

Can complications occur?

There are no complications associated with lung function tests.

Further reading

Armstrong P and Wastie M (1981) X-ray Diagnosis, Blackwell Scientific

Belcher J and Sturridge M (1972) Thoracic Surgery Management, 4th edition, Baillière Tindall

Brewis R (1980) Lecture Notes on Respiratory Disease, Blackwell Scientific

Cameron T (1981) Fibreoptic bronchoscopy, American Journal of Nursing 81: 1942–1944

Chesney D and Chesney M (1978) Care of the Patient During Radiological Procedures, Blackwell Scientific

Cotes J (1979) Lung Function, 4th edition, Blackwell Scientific

Fream W (1978) Notes on Surgical Nursing, 2nd edition, Churchill Livingstone

Grenville Mathers R (1976) Respiratory System, Churchill Livingstone

Sproule S (1981) Fundamentals of Respiratory Disease, Blackwell Scientific

CHAPTER 8

INVESTIGATIONS ASSOCIATED WITH THE URINARY TRACT

The renal or urinary system consists of two kidneys each with a ureter opening into the bladder. The bladder opens onto the exterior by the urethra. The functions of this system are to maintain homoeostasis and to produce urine in which excess water and waste products of metabolism can be excreted from the body.

Disease or trauma to any part of this system may interfere with the normal function of the system and the body as a whole.

Investigations associated with this system are often complex and time-consuming. They may also be potentially embarrassing for the patient. Nurses and other staff involved should empathize with the patient, give clear explanations and be very precise in the preparations that are made and in the care which is given.

8.1   Renal Arteriogram

What is a renal arteriogram?

This is an investigation where radio-opaque dye is injected into the aorta just above the renal arteries to show the arterial pattern of both kidneys.

Why is a renal arteriogram performed?

1   To confirm stenosis of the renal artery or one of its branches.

2   To differentiate between a carcinoma or a cyst in the kidney (a carcinoma would have its own blood supply).

3   To confirm death of a kidney.

4   The investigation is also sometimes used when there has been abdominal trauma to aid the surgeon to see whether it is either safe or necessary for surgical intervention.

112

Where is the renal arteriogram performed and what preparation is necessary?

A renal arteriogram is an invasive procedure and does carry a degree of risk. Careful explanation is important. It is necessary for the patient to sign a consent form for this procedure, so the doctor must ensure that the patient is fully aware of what it entails before he signs. Sometimes a lumbar approach is used, which entails a general anaesthetic. The femoral approach only will be considered here.

The day before the investigation the right groin should be shaved to prevent any infection from the hair. An iodine patch test should also be carried out to ensure that the patient is not sensitive to the dye. The patient should have nothing to eat or drink for 6 hours prior to the test, and should have a bath, possibly using an antiseptic solution (depending upon hospital policy). The patient should wear a hospital gown for the test. False teeth, glasses and jewellery should be removed. The patient is asked to empty his bladder. In some cases a premedication is given.   This ensures that the patient is as relaxed as possible.

How is a renal arteriogram performed?

This procedure is carried out in the X-ray department. The patient arrives in the department on a trolley, accompanied by a nurse. The patient is transferred onto the investigation table and is secured with wide straps. These are necessary as the table is tipped to disperse the dye and to enable pictures to be taken from all angles. The doctor performing the procedure and the nurse assisting are gowned up as for theatre, and will clean the groin area with an antiseptic solution. They will then drape the patient in sterile towels to create a sterile working area. Some local anaesthetic is injected into the groin — a stinging sensation may occur — and time allowed for it to work. A femoral arterial stab is then performed — pressure will be felt — and a catheter passed along the arteries until the point in the aorta just above the renal arteries is reached. Dye is then injected into the catheter and pictures are taken of its course around the renal arteries. The injection of the dye may give the patient a hot, flushed feeling, but this should pass. The procedure should not be painful, the patient should only be able to feel the pressure of the catheter.

When the dye has been injected and the pictures taken the catheter is removed. Firm pressure is applied to the wound site until it has stopped bleeding, for 10 min at least. The wound is not sutured — a small dressing is applied. The patient is now ready to return to the ward. A nurse should accompany the patient.

What happens after the renal arteriogram?

Because the wound is in a major vessel and not sutured, the patient has to stay in bed for 24 hours trying to move the leg as little as possible. He will therefore need help with washing, urinals or bedpans. Make sure everything on his locker is within easy reach. The patient can eat or drink as soon as he is fully awake, starting slowly with sips of water.

Half-hourly observations of blood pressure, the wound site and the pulse for signs of a haemorrhage, colour and sensation of the foot on the affected side should be made at first, to identify any circulatory abnormality. These can become less frequent as the patient's condition stabilizes.

When are the results available and what might they be?

The radiologist will report on the X-rays and the doctor should have the final report within 48 hours. Possible findings include:

1   Stenosis of the renal artery or one of its branches
2   Renal cyst or carcinoma.
3   Renal death.
4   Trauma to the kidney.

Contraindications for a renal anteriogram

There are no contraindications

Can complications occur?

Complications occasionally occur:

1   Allergic reaction to the dye. A test dose should always be given prior to the full dose.
2   Haemorrhage — from the wound site. This is why frequent close observation is carried out. Firm pressure will have to be applied to the site if haemorrhage does occur and the doctor informed.
3   Embolism — emboli may be dislodged by the catheter.

8.2.   Intravenous Pyelogram (IVP) (Urogram)

What is an intravenous pyelogram (IVP)?

An intravenous pyelogram is an X-ray investigation using radio-opaque medium to obtain a complete picture of the upper urinary tract. It shows the kidneys, ureters and bladder.

Why is an intravenous pyelogram performed?

The investigation is performed to see the position, symmetry and size of the kidneys, the anatomy of the renal calyces and pelvis, and to see the course of each ureter. The investigation may be performed to discover the cause of any suspected renal disease.

An IVP is a very common investigation and can show many things. Some of the more common findings include renal or ureteric calculi; an enlarged prostate gland, polycystic kidneys; renal tuberculosis or a nonfunctioning kidney; or tumours.

Where is the intravenous pyelogram performed and what preparation is necessary?

The investigation is carried out in the X-ray department. Explanation is very important. A clear bowel is also essential if a clear picture of the upper urinary tract is to be seen. An aperient should be given to the patient the night before, and a phosphate enema on the day of the investigation. The patient should have no fluids for 3–4 hours before the investigation. This is to ensure that the dye is more concentrated and will show up clearly on the X-ray. The patient may eat normally, but because of the fluid restriction, a dry breakfast may be necessary. A bath and clean hospital gown will reduce the risk of infection. All jewellery and glasses should be removed.

The investigation is not painful. Some people, however, do feel a hot flush as the dye is injected into the vein, whilst others get a taste of onions in their mouth. The patient should be warned that these may occur.

How is the intravenous pyelogram performed?

The patient lies on a table and a small test dose of dye is injected intravenously by the doctor. If the patient shows no abnormal reaction to the dye 20–40 ml are injected into a vein in the arm. The dye is excreted from the body by the kidney, so X-ray photographs taken at intervals will show its passage through the upper urinary tract. The X-rays are usually taken after 5-, 15- and 30-min intervals. After the last X-ray the procedure is over, and the patient may return to the ward.

What happens after the intravenous pyelogram?

Ask the patient how the investigation went. The patient may now drink normally. The injection site should be checked to ensure that it is not bleeding. Close observation of the patient will detect delayed reaction to the dye. Indications of this would be a rash, the patient feeling hot, giddy or faint or any other abnormal feeling.

When are the results available and what might they be?

It is sometimes possible to tell the patient the results immediately, but there is often a delay of 24–48 hours while the radiologist reports on the X-rays. Possible findings include:

1   Renal or ureteric calculi.

2   An enlarged prostate gland.

3   Polycystic kidneys.

4   Renal tuberculosis.

5   A nonfunctioning kidney.

6   Tumours.

Contraindications for an intravenous pyelogram

The investigation is usually contraindicated during pregnancy and in advanced chronic renal failure. There is some evidence to suggest that when Bence Jones protein is present in the urine, an IVP may precipitate an attack of acute renal failure.

Can complications occur?

Complications may include:

1   A reaction to the contrast medium, which may lead to anaphylactic shock. An adrenalin injection is always prepared in case of this emergency.

2   Bleeding, or infection of the injection site.

Patients' comments

'I felt a little squeamish, but no pain at all. Doctor explained it well to me and I knew it was to see the kidneys and ureters and my bladder. They took many X-rays, but I couldn't see enough myself of what the X-rays showed. They like to wait for the consultant to see them I kept asking questions and so knew what it was all about. Quite simple really!'

'When the doctor put the needle into my arm and injected the dye, it made me feel hot between the ears, but it passed off in a few minutes. The doctor told me that this always happened and it was the dye going round my body to my bladder.'

'The dye made my head feel like a boomerang, but it soon felt better. I had to lie flat on the table for the X-rays, and had to breath in and out. It took about ¾ hour. I felt a little sick when I came back, but rested on my bed and soon felt better.'

8.3.   Renal Biopsy

What is a renal biopsy?

A renal biopsy is where a small portion of kidney tissue is obtained with a puncture needle for histology.

Why is a renal biopsy performed?

A renal biopsy is used to confirm the nature of kidney disease when the diagnosis cannot be made by other means.

Where is the renal biopsy performed and what preparation is necessary?

Renal biopsy is usually performed in the ward. In order for a renal biopsy to be performed the patient should have two functioning kidneys and no bleeding disorders or kidney infection. Before the biopsy is performed an intravenous pyelogram (see Section 8.2) is carried out to establish the position of the kidneys. A simple and clear explanation is given to the patient to help ensure cooperation. Privacy and dignity should be maintained. The patient should empty his bladder prior to the procedure. A sterile trolley is prepared as per hospital procedure.

How is the renal biopsy performed?

The positioning of the patient is important so that the correct position of the kidneys can be located. The patient lies in the prone position with a sandbag under the abdomen. The position of the kidney is marked using the boney landmarks and measurements from the intravenous pyelogram. A strict aspetic technique is used and the area is cleaned with sterile swabs. Local anaesthetic is then injected into the appropriate area. The patient may feel the initial injection of local anaesthetic and then only a 'pressure' feeling as the biopsy needle is introduced. The kidney tissue is collected with a renal puncture needle. The tissue specimen is put into a specimen pot in a fixative, labelled and sent to the laboratory for histology. The puncture site has an occlusive dressing applied. This can be removed after 48 hours.

What happens after the renal biopsy?

The patient is kept in the prone position for 30 min to maintain pressure on the kidney and minimize bleeding. Observations of pulse and blood pressure are made $\frac{1}{2}$–2-hourly until stable, and all urine is tested for blood. This is to ensure early detection of signs of internal haemorrhage. The patient is kept in bed to rest for 24 hours to minimize the risk of bleeding. The patient should be warned that he may have haematuria. He can eat and drink as normal.

When are the results available and what might they be?

A report on the biopsy may take a few days. Possible findings include:

1   Renal disease.
2   Renal infection.
3   Malignant disease.

Contraindications for renal biopsy

1   Nonfunctioning kidney or kidneys.
2   Bleeding disorders.
3   Renal infection.

Can complications occur?

Haemorrhage, which might be indicated by backache, shoulder pain or dysuria. The doctor should be informed immediately.

8.4.   Videocystogram and Micturating Cystograms

What are video- and micturating cystograms?

These are X-ray investigations using a radio-opaque medium to observe the functioning of the bladder. The pressures both inside and outside the bladder are monitored whilst it is filling and emptying. The pressures are monitored on a graph and the filling of the bladder can be seen on a television screen. The effectiveness of the internal and external sphincters can also be observed.

Why are video- and micturating cystograms performed?

This investigation is usually performed to determine the cause of a poor or abnormal micturating pattern. The investigation will show several defects if present — including an atonic bladder, bladder tumours, incontinence (and sometimes the cause of it) and vesico-ureteric reflux.

Where are video- and micturating cystograms performed and what preparation is necessary?

The cystogram is performed in the X-ray department. This is an embarrassing and unpleasant investigation, so a careful explanation of the procedure is essential. The patient should be warned that he will be asked to pass urine whilst several people, often of both sexes, are watching him. He should be reassured as far as possible that the doctors and nurses have seen many before and do understand his embarrassment. The patient should also be told that the investigation is not painful but the small wire probe introduced into the rectum may be uncomfortable.

The doctors often want to take a flow rate from the patient before the investigation, and it is therefore helpful if he can attend with a full bladder. The patient should be wearing a hospital gown, but there may be some waiting around so advise him to take a dressing gown and a book. Jewellery should be removed and stored safely.

How are video- and micturating cystograms performed?

When the patient arrives in the X-ray room he will be asked to pass urine so that the flow rate can be obtained. This is not particularly embarrassing as it is just the same as passing urine normally, with nobody watching — a special toilet is used and the patient may be asked to press a button when they start and finish micturating.

The patient will then be helped onto a table and asked to lie on his left-hand side. A fine rectal wire is introduced, which measures the pressure inside the rectum, and at the back of the bladder. This is uncomfortable but not painful. The bladder is filled with the radio-opaque solution which is run in from an intravenous infusion set via a catheter that has been introduced into the bladder via the urethra. The patient is asked to say when he feels that his bladder is full, or when he feels uncomfortable. The amount of fluid in the bladder is measured and the filling process watched on a television screen. The investigation up to this point is called a videocystogram.

The table is tilted upwards until the patient is standing in a vertical position. He is asked to relax and allow the fluid in his bladder to flow back into the bag. The pressures are measured as the patient micturates. The fluid is then run back into the bladder and the catheter removed. The patient is then asked to pass the fluid into a funnel-shaped piece of apparatus.

After the investigation the doctor may reintroduce the catheter to drain off any fluid that the patient has been unable to pass. At any time throughout the procedure the patient may be asked to stop passing water in midstream, or to cough. All this is to assess the function of the bladder as fully as possible. The pressures throughout are recorded on a graph, and the filling and emptying of the bladder can be seen on a television screen. The catheter will be removed and the patient can return to the ward.

What happens after video- and micturating cystograms

Ask how the investigation went. The nurse should warn the patient that his urine may be bloodstained. Oral fluids should be encouraged — about 1 litre in 12 hours following the investigation — to ensure that all the dye is flushed out of the bladder. Urine output should be recorded for 24 hours at least.

When are the results available and what might they be?

The results should be available within 2–3 days. Possible findings include:

1   Atonic bladder.

2   Bladder tumour.

3   Incontinence.

4   Vesicoureteric reflux.

Contraindications for video- and micturating cystograms

This procedure requires a high degree of patient cooperation, so it may be inappropriate for confused or uncooperative patients.

Can complications occur?

Complications include the introduction of a urinary tract infection, cystitis, haemorrhage and damage to the urethra or bladder. All these are rare and in most cases avoidable, but the nurse should be aware of them.

Patients' comments

'I had to drink gallons before I had the investigation. The doctor told me about it, that it was to see my bladder and to measure the pressure of what came out. I had to pass water as they watched a telly screen. It was difficult to go with all the nurses around, but really I wasn't very worried about who was there, I knew I had to go to get a good result, and so I made myself get on with it.'

'Before the X-ray I had to drink lots. I found it rather humiliating and dramatic passing urine in the room with the operators, and I did feel a little poked around. But that is what it is all about and it had to be done to get the best proper result.'

8.5.   Twenty-four-hourly Urine Collections

Twenty-four-hourly urine collections may be used to assess kidney function or to measure a certain waste product, e.g., creatinine, which may be present in the urine and so indicate of impaired renal function.

How is the 24-hourly urine collection performed?

The bladder is emptied and the urine discarded immediately before commencing the 24-hour collection. During the following 24 hours all urine passed must be collected in the appropriate container. If a specimen is discarded the collection needs to be restarted. At the end of the 24-hour period the bladder is emptied and this is added to the collection. If the collection is not to be sent immediately to the laboratory it must be kept in a specimen refrigerator. It must be ensured that the correct container and preservative are used for specific tests, and also that the patient uses a clean receptacle into which to pass the urine.

What is a creatinine clearance test?

Creatinine clearance is a test to assess renal function. A 24-hour collection of urine is made in a suitable container containing methiolate preservative. Clotted blood, 10 ml, has to be taken at some time during the 24 hours. It is a measure of the volume of blood cleared of creatinine in 1 min. Normally this is 70–130 ml/min. This is related to body area and so the result has to be multiplied by a correction factor for children and obese adults. The normal daily excretion of creatinine is about 10 mmol for a woman and 20 mmol for a man.

8.6.   Midstream Specimen of Urine (MSSU)

What is a midstream specimen of urine?

A midstream specimen of urine is that part of a specimen collected halfway through micturation so that the specimen is less contaminated.

Why is a midstream specimen of urine collected?

The specimen is sent for culture and sensitivity testing:

1   To confirm a urinary tract infection.
2   To confirm the presence of malignant cells.

How is a midstream specimen of urine collected?

For accurate results to be obtained the specimen collected should be as free from outside contamination as possible. The genital area should be washed well using soap and water, so that it is socially clean, and dried with a clean towel. The procedure is explained to the patient who will carry it out himself. If he is unable to, the nurse will carry out the procedure for him. Absolute privacy and plenty of time is essential if a specimen is to be obtained, particularly if the nurse is carrying out the procedure.

In the case of male patients the end of the penis and the foreskin should be carefully cleaned using sterile swabs and a sterile lotion, e.g., normal saline which will not contaminate the specimen. For female patients the labia minora and the urethral orifice are cleaned — one swab being used once, moving away from the clean area. If possible the cleaned labia should be held apart during micturition, a disposable glove being provided to protect the patient's hand.

The patient begins to pass urine into the toilet, bedpan or urinal, then stops and passes the midstream specimen of about 40–60 ml into a sterile container. Once this is collected the patient can continue to empty the bladder normally. The specimen should be in a sterile container with an airtight lid. It should be labelled and sent with the pathological request form to the laboratory as soon as possible.

NOTE: If a patient is menstruating this may contaminate the specimen and the fact should be recorded on the pathology request form.

8.7. Early Morning Urine specimen (EMUS)

Why is an early morning urine specimen (EMUS) collected?

An early morning specimen is usually collected to determine whether the patient is suffering from renal tuberculosis. Three EMUS's are usually sent on consecutive mornings.

How is an early morning urine specimen collected?

The genital area is cleaned in the normal way using soap and water then the whole of the specimen is collected. This should be the first urine that the person passes on waking. As urine contains substances that destroy the tubercule bacillus on standing, the urine samples must be sent over to the laboratory as soon as possible each day. This specimen is also collected to confirm pregnancy.

Further reading

Cameron S (1981) Kidney Diseases: The Facts, OUP

Cameron S (1976) Nephrology for Nurses, 2nd edition, Heinemann Medical

Chapman S and Nakielny R (1981) Guide to Radiological Procedures, Baillière Tindall

Chilman A and Thomas M (1981) Understanding Nursing Care, 2nd edition, Churchill Livingstone

Gabriel R (1981) Renal Medicine, Baillière Tindall

Jameson R (1976) Management of Urology Patient, Churchill Livingstone

McConnell E (1981) Urinalysis: common but never routine, Nursing (US) 11: 8–9

McGuckin M (1981) Getting better urine specimens with clean-catch midstream technique, Nursing (US) 11: 72–73

Mitchell J (1981) Urology for Nurses, 3rd edition, John Wright

Newsam J and Petrie J (1978) Urology and Renal Medicine, 3rd edition, Churchill Livingstone

Uldall R (1977) Renal Nursing, 2nd edition, Blackwell Scientific

CHAPTER 9

MISCELLANEOUS INVESTIGATION PROCEDURES

Included in this short section are investigations which might be used on any system and involve new technology and large, potentially frightening equipment.

9.1. Computerized Axial Tomography (CT Scan)

What is computerized axial tomography (CT scan)?

The CT scan allows the relationships and densities of a patient's anatomy to be seen, by producing an image of a transverse slice through the patient at a given level within the body. Any abnormalities, such as a tumour, can therefore be detected. The CT scanner employs conventional X-rays, which are more sophisticated, showing more detail of the internal organs, their contents and much soft tissue, as well as bone. Instead of using a film to produce the information, a computer reproduces the patient's anatomy as a picture.

Why is a CT scan performed?

There are two main reasons for doing this investigation:

To identify the size, shape and position of the organs and structures in the abdomen. For example:

1   Splenic enlargement.
2   Liver metastases.
3   Enlarged abdominal lymph glands.
4   Enlarged pancreas.
5   Abdominal masses.

To identify the anatomy of the brain for diagnostic purposes. For example:

1   Cerebral vascular accident.

2   Infarcts.

3   Metastases.

4   Neurofibromas.

5   Tumours.

Where is the CT scan performed and what preparation is necessary?

All patients have nothing to eat for 4 hours before scanning. A cup of tea or coffee is allowed.

Abdominal scans

1   Patients must follow a low residue diet for 2 days prior to the investigation.
    a. Suitable foods: lean meat, grilled fish, steamed vegetables, creamed potatoes, custard, jelly, milk pudding.
    b. Unsuitable foods: green vegetables, citrus fruits, apples, toast, baked beans, fatty foods, salads.

2   At least 2 pints of fluid must be taken in the form of water, tea, coffee, milk or cordial. Fizzy drinks must not be taken.

3   Nothing is eaten on the day of the investigation, but drinks of tea, coffee or squash are permitted.

4   Laxatives must NOT be taken. This is important, because they reduce the amount of gas in the bowel, which would prevent seeing clear pictures, and also reduce the movement of the bowel which would give distorted pictures.

How is the CT scan performed?

The CT scan is a relatively harmless investigation used to visualize the internal organs instead of a major investigative operation. The machine is large, and through the middle is a short tunnel. A long couch on a movable trolley runs through this tunnel and may be adjusted to the correct position for each part of the body to be scanned. Around the tunnel, hidden by metal, are the X-ray beams which take the pictures. So the part of the body in the tunnel is X-rayed. Each scan takes about 20 s but many pictures are needed to give a realistic, clear result. There is a slight noise from the machine as the pictures are taken, but nothing to be alarmed about. The complete scanning takes about 40 min.

Head scans   The patient is asked to lie on the couch, when an injection of iodine-based contrast medium is injected into the arm, e.g., 60 ml of Conray 420 intravenously. This is to show the blood supply. The contrast medium travels around the body, and the blood vessels in the head are clearly defined on the X-ray. A doctor must give this injection.

Bean bags are placed on either side of the patient's head to keep it still during X-ray. The radiographer then operates the couch and moves it backwards so that the head is in the tunnel. The radiographer leaves the room and takes the X-rays via a computer in an adjacent room. However, the radiographer talks to the patient through a microphone and can clearly see and hear the patient the whole time.

Abdominal scans   The patient is asked to drink a solution of contrast medium, e.g., Gastrografin 5%, 300–400 ml. This gives the small bowel a higher density than the organs, and therefore gives a clearer picture. Side-effects are allergies and nausea. This solution has an aniseed flavour. The patient then lies on the couch and the X-rays are taken. The patient is asked to hold his breath (this is to displace the organs from beneath the diaphragm to give a clearer picture). If there is considerable activity of the bowel and the pictures are not clear, a doctor may give Buscopan 20 mg in 1 ml intravenously to reduce this movement.

What happens after the CT scan?

There is no specific aftercare. The patient may eat and drink normally.

When are the results available and what might they be?

It may take a few days to analyse the films. Possible findings include:

1   Neoplasms.
2   Metastases.
3   Abdominal masses.
4   Infarctions.

Contraindications for CT scans

There are no contraindications.

Can complications occur?

There are no complications.

Patients' comments

'It was like sitting inside an automatic washing machine. There was a round port hole in which I put my head. I must add the washing machine was not going round and round!'

'I put my head in a tunnel and the staff positioned me very comfortably with foam pads around my head. They made sure my back was comfortable before leaving me. They were in the room next door, but there was a microphone, so I could hear them and they could hear me. They kept asking me whether I was alright!'

'Shame you can't see anything while the pictures are taken. It is a lonely feeling, but they played the radio to me. They spent 20 min taking pictures. The tunnel around your head clicks away and you hear things moving, but it isn't frightening. Then a dye was put in my arm. This was a peculiar feeling. It was like being 'topped up' with something warm, but not unpleasant. This warmth went up and down my body for a couple of minutes and then 20 min more of pictures were taken. After the investigation when I bent forwards the same vague feelings of warmth in my head happened for about 6 hours. Anyway, I knew what to expect and so it wasn't so bad.'

9.2.   Ultrasound

What is Ultrasound?

Ultrasound is a diagnostic procedure employing high-frequency sound waves, high above the range of human audition. It is used to map the echoes from regions of tissues where changes in sound properties occur, and thus in ultrasound there is reliance principally on the elastic density properties of materials. Special devices, called transducers, are needed to induce vibrations at these high frequencies. The ultrasound waves pass through the body and are reflected at the various interfaces and particle boundaries. Usually in medicine the same transducer is used as both the transmitter and receiver of the ultrasound waves. The images thus received are produced as thin slices or tomograms, which represent the distribution of tissues, and are the acoustic (hearing) representation of these structures. These images appear on a television screen via a computer.

Ultrasound is safer than radiography since it does not use ionizing radiation. A main area of application is in obstetrics for routine investigations of foetal growth, when radiography is particularly dangerous. Ultrasound is relatively simple to perform, and safe. The technology is relatively cheap, and it is therefore suitable for population screening. As a diagnostic tool its use is growing continuously. This is due to both improvements in equipment design and the interpretation of the displayed information.

Why is ultrasound performed?

Ultrasound scanning is valuable in differentiating tumour deposits from abscesses or cysts, as this method can show if a lesion is solid or if it contains fluid.

Ultrasound is used in obstetrics to demonstrate or monitor:

1   Foetal size and growth.

2   Number of foetuses and presentation.

3   Position of placenta.

4   Obstetric problems, e.g., hydatidiform mole, ectopic pregnancy.

5   Amniocentesis, e.g., taking a specimen of the amniotic fluid to be examined as a guide for the condition of an unborn baby. The needle is guided through the abdominal wall with the help of the ultrasound which indicates the position of the baby in relation to the needle. At present only a few congenital diseases, such as Down's syndrome, can be recognized in this way. However, the technique is developing fast and in the future other chromosome abnormalities will be able to be detected.

Ultrasound is used in gynaecology to:

1   Demonstrate the presence and nature of pelvic masses.

2   Check ultrauterine devices, e.g., coil correctly positioned.

Ultrasound is used in urology to demonstrate:

1   Presence and nature of pelvic masses.

2   Renal size and shape.

3   Space occupying legions in kidney.

4   Hydronephrosis.

Ultrasound is used in gastroenterology to demonstrate:

1   Calibre of biliary tree for differential diagnosis of jaundice.

2   Pancreatic disease.

3   Gall stones.

4   Associated liver problems.

5   Gastric lesions, e.g., cancer may sometimes be demonstrated if *large* (but barium and X-ray investigations are still best for gut).

Use on thyroid: to detect and comment on lumps in the neck. Thyroid cysts may be aspirated under ultrasonic control.

Use on breast: to detect differences between solid and cystic lumps. As techniques improve, ultrasound may be used for screening purposes.

Use on limbs: to identify tissue swellings and to discover whether they consist of blood or tissue fluid.

Use on head: limited–superseded by the CT scan. However, it is used in neonates through the anterior fontanelle.

Use in cardiology: to demonstrate heart-valve motion, pericardial effusions, etc.

Where is ultrasound performed and what preparation is necessary?

Ultrasound is harmless and painless and no preparation is required, except for pelvic and abdominal scans. The scanning does not take long, since a single image is accumulated in a few seconds, and most examinations take 15–20 min to complete. Results from the ultrasound may be immediate, but depending upon the type of scan and clarity of the picture, the results may not be available until the pictures have been studied and assessed.

Pelvic scan   The bladder must be *full*, since it provides a good 'acoustic window' into the pelvis, and enables the ultrasonographer to see more clearly into the pelvis. The patient should drink 1–1½ litres of water 1 hour before scanning.

Abdominal scan   As little air as possible must be in the gut, because ultrasound does not travel through air, and no pictures can be taken. So the patient should have nothing to eat or drink 6 hours before the scan.

Gall bladder investigations   Smoking may cause contraction of the gall bladder, so it is advisable not to smoke before the investigation.

How is ultrasound performed?

An appointment system is used, and the patient should be seen on time, so they should be properly prepared (especially for pelvic scans). The patient is asked to change into a white gown, and to lie on a couch. The site to be scanned is exposed, and oil is placed over this area to provide good contact between the probe and the skin. Sound waves do not travel through air. The ultrasonographer then begins to move the probe back and forth in a sweeping movement over the skin. Quite quickly the picture is seen on the screen. With abdominal scans the patient is asked to take a deep breath in and hold it. This displaces the organs from under the rib cage for a better picture. When the scan is completed, the skin is cleaned and the patient may resume normal activities.

What happens after ultrasound?

There is no specific aftercare. The patient may eat and drink normally.

When are the results available and what might they be?

Results are available immediately in most cases.

Contraindications for ultrasound

There are no contraindications for ultrasound

Can complications occur?

There are no complications associated with ultrasound.

Patients' comments

'The most exciting experience of my life. I didn't know what was going to happen, but she explained it all very well. I felt really feminine — seeing the baby on the screen. I was not concerned about the procedure — my whole interest was directed to the screen.'

'I was amazed that the ultrasound was able to give the doctors such a clear view of the internal organs of my body.'

'The doctors told me that this ultrasound saved me from having many painful investigations and even operations.'

'I had a pelvic scan and the nurses on my ward told me to drink so much water. I was nearly bursting, but I know that better pictures are taken if you have drunk lots.'

'It was so easy and simple. Nothing to be worried about. I'd go again any day.'

9.3.   Radiological Investigations

Many investigations involving radiological techniques are included in the individual systems sections. In this section some of the main facts have been brought together.

What is an X-ray?

An X-ray is an electromagnetic ray which can penetrate solid substances and enable photographs to be taken of internal organs. The equipment used is often large and complex and this can cause the patient most anxiety when X-rays are being performed. Clear explanation must therefore be given about the equipment as well as the procedure.

Why is an X-ray performed?

X-rays are taken to confirm or aid diagnosis. Plain X-rays visualize solid structures like bones. It is necessary to use some form of contrast medium to visualize soft tissues and organs.

Where is the X-ray performed and what preparation is necessary?

X-rays are commonly taken in the radiology department, but can be taken in the ward if the patient is too ill to be moved, or in theatre during surgery. Mobile equipment is used. X-rays can also be carried out on an outpatient basis.

    Little preparation is required for X-rays such as chest X-rays or skeletal X-rays, but for others very precise preparation is necessary. Reference should be made to the X-ray department regarding this. However, certain basic points should be remembered. All jewellery or metal objects, such as hair grips, should be removed from the field that is going to be X-rayed as their image may mask something on the X-ray. A gown with no buttons should be worn — this again gives a clear field. Previous X-rays should accompany the patient to the department as they may be used for comparison.

NOTE: For specific procedures and aftercare, see the individual investigations.

When are the results available and what might they be?

Major abnormalities can be seen immediately the film is developed, but more detailed reporting will take a day or two.

Contraindications for an X-ray

Contraindications for an X-ray include allergic reaction to contrast medium used. If anaesthesia is involved, either local or general, there may be complications. Prophylaxis to avoid adverse reactions includes pretesting with contrast medium, pretreatment with steroids for those who have previously had severe adverse reaction or those at risk.

Can complications occur?

All radiological procedures carry some degree of risk because ionized radiation is used. Rapidly dividing cells are most vulnerable, therefore X-rays of a female's pelvis during her 'reproductive life' are carried out very carefully and only if absolutely necessary. A 10 day rule has been devised.

The 10-day rule (RCR 1976)   This applies to examination of the lower abdomen (nipples to knees) of all female patients of reproductive capacity (12–50 years) and should be carried out within 10 days following the first day of the menstrual cycle. Exceptions to this are:

1   Women who deny recent sexual intercourse.

2   Women who are menstruating.

3   Women who have been taking the contraceptive pill for no less than 3 months.

4   Women with intrauterine contraceptive devices in situ for no less than 3 months.

5   Women who have been sterilized.

Women in the first trimester of pregnancy will only be X-rayed in an emergency because of risk to the developing foetus.

Further Reading

Armstrong P and Wastie M (1981) X-Ray Diagnosis, Blackwell Scientific

Brackenridge R (1979) Essential Medicine, 2nd edition, MTP

Chapman S and Nakielny R (1981) Guide to Radiological Procedures, Baillière Tindall

Donald L (1981) All in a day's work: role of the trained nurse in CT unit, Nursing Mirror 152: 44

Haughey C (1981) Understanding ultrasonography, Nursing (US) 11: 34–35

Husband J and Golding S (1982) Computed tomography of the body: when it should be used, British Medical Journal 284: 224–228

MacLeod J (editor) (1981) Davidson's Principles and Practice of Medicine, 13th edition, Churchill Livingstone

Nash D (1980) Principles and Practice of Surgery for Nurses and Allied Professionals, 7th edition, Edward Arnold

Valentine A (1981) Practical Introduction to Cranial CT, Heinemann Medical

Other titles in the **Lippincott Nursing Series**

SI Units for Nurses, by John Glenn, British Campus, University of Evansville, and David McCaugherty, Tutor, School of Nursing, Princess Margaret Hospital, Swindon.

Legal Problems in Nursing Practice, by Ann Young, Senior Tutor, Thomas Guy School of Nursing, Guy's Hospital, London.

Lippincott Manual of Paediatric Nursing, by Lillian S Brunner and Doris S Suddarth, adapted for the UK by Barbara Weller.

Physiology in Nursing, by Marguerita Brunt, Senior Tutor (Postbasis Education), Hammersmith Hospital School of Nursing, London.

Communication for the Health Care Team, by Voncile M Smith and Thelma A Bass, adapted for the UK by Ann Faulkner.

Patient Related Multiple Choice Questions by Anne Betts, Cynthia Gilling, Marjorie Read and Maureen Theobald, Princess Alexandra School of Nursing, The London Hospital, London.
Book 1 — The Patient with a Respiratory Disorder
Book 2 — The Patient with a Cardiovascular Disorder.

The Lippincott Manual of Medical-Surgical Nursing, Volumes 1, 2 and 3, by Lillian S Brunner and Doris S Suddarth, Adapted for the UK.